LOOKING GOOD

A comprehensive guide to wardrobe planning, color & personal style development.

by Nancy Nix-Rice

Editor and photographer: Pati Palmer
Designer: Linda Wisner
Image Consultant and Stylist: Ethel Harms
Illustrators: Diane Russell, Kate Pryka
and Jeannette Schilling

A *Palmer/Pletsch*
PUBLICATION

I've always questioned the sincerity of authors who say "No book is the work of a single person"... but now I understand exactly what they mean. *Looking Good* would never exist without the help of countless other talented people:

- Leslie Wood and Barbara Weiland, whose earlier book *Clothes Sense* inspired this book.
- The publisher, Pati Palmer, who artfully brought all the pieces together... and who also became the photographer.
- Design director Linda Wisner, who turned my words into these exciting, easy-to-read pages.
- Design assistant Jeannette Schilling, who in addition to her technical and artistic contributions, was a wonderful sport about posing for the dramatic before and after photos on page 6, allowing us to select the distinctly unflattering clothing and pose for her "before" photo.
- Artists Diane Kramer and Kate Pryka, who made each concept so vividly visual.
- Image consultant Ethel Harms, who influenced the look of the photography.
- The models, who beautifully demonstrated the concepts in this book.
- Carolyn Olson, whose classes vastly improved my writing style.
- And Ann Price Gosch, who provided positive feedback while she fine-tuned the grammar and construction.

The information in this book isn't new or revolutionary. It is time-tested and proven by hundreds of image consultants, many of whom have generously shared their knowledge with me over the years:

- Susan Bixler, author and president of Professional Image Institute
- Norma Virgin of Beauty for All Seasons
- Karla Jordan and Julie Mucha of Karla Jordan International
- Georgia Palmer, CK Reisinger and Sally Ellston of Doncaster
- Mary Marcdante and Carla Kay, whose presentations many years ago convinced me that I wanted to be an image consultant "when I grew up"

This book is lovingly dedicated to my mother and my "other mother" Edith, both of whom taught me to appreciate loveliness both external and internal, and to my daughters Mandy and Katie, for their joy in learning those same lessons all over again.

Whenever brand names are mentioned, it is only to indicate to the consumer products which we have personally tested and with which we have been pleased. It is also meant to save our students time. There may be other products that are comparable to aid you.

Cover art by Diane Russell.

Copyright © 1996 by Palmer/Pletsch Incorporated. Third printing 1998.
Library of Congress Catalog Card Number: 97-78484
Published by Palmer/Pletsch Publishing, P.O. Box 12046, Portland, OR 97212-0046. U.S.A.
Printed by Craftsman Press, Seattle, WA, U.S.A. Separations and film work by Wy'East, Portland, OR.

ISBN 0-935278-42-7

Table of Contents

Foreword by Pati Palmer

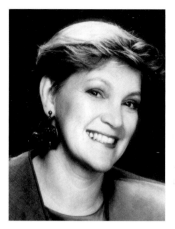

Our first image book, *Clothes Sense*, by home economists Leslie Wood and Barbara Weiland, was lauded as the most comprehensive book ever written about wardrobe planning when we published it in 1984. Packed with design theory, realistic examples and illustrations, it remained a favorite of image consultants for more than a decade.

As times changed, though—

- readers came to expect color in books—especially in visual subjects like image and wardrobe;
- theories of personal coloring grew more sophisticated;
- garment styles evolved toward the casual;
- technology developed exciting new fabrics;
- women's lifestyles moved in new directions; and
- the population aged.

In short, it was time for a beautiful, new, color volume about wardrobe planning.

Nancy Nix-Rice, an image consultant with a life-long involvement in the fashion-sewing industry, approached us with an offer to update and expand *Clothes Sense*. And, with the blessing of the original authors, that gem of a book became the foundation and inspiration for the new *Looking Good*.

The book is about you—a REAL woman—and the daily challenges you face looking good while you juggle all the other aspects of your busy life. We didn't use tall, willowy models to illustrate our advice—we used **real people**.

- One make-over was a gift to our design assistant, Jeannette Schilling. The change was so dramatic that when we went to meet her for lunch later that day, we walked right by her!

- My sister-in-law Marty Palmer, a fuller figure, often wears an overblouse the way many of us do, to hide the middle. Just a few changes convinced us all there is a better way.

- Even I accepted a modeling assignment and proved that tucking in an overblouse, on a full-hipped figure, can indeed be more flattering. We all gasped when we saw the first before and after Polaroids. It was quite an eye-opener.

For the photography sessions, we recruited professional image consultant and stylist Ethel Harms to help with hair, makeup and clothing. We scrupulously avoided any photographic "tricks." You know the kind—harsh lighting used for the "befores" and softly tinted, filtered lighting to enhance the "afters." Instead, our film and lighting were as natural as they could be...so the changes you see are REAL!

We also avoided labeling any choices as RIGHT or WRONG, GOOD or BAD. Beauty is in the eyes of the beholder, and each woman has her own unique "raw material," wardrobe objectives, and personal priorities. We do point out the choices that our experience has shown to be more pleasing. Our photography illustrates those concepts for you to assess and apply.

Get involved with the book. As you complete each exercise—from the Personal Style quiz to the Closet Clean-out and the Capsule Wardrobe plan—we believe you will discover a more beautiful, more confident you. Your closet will be more organized and your wardrobe dollars invested more wisely.

We hope you will enjoy LOOKING GOOD.

Pati Palmer

Owner and CEO
Palmer/Pletsch Publishing

About the Author

Nancy Nix-Rice is a wardrobe and image consultant for women and men from homemakers and preschool teachers to corporate executives and television personalities. Her home-based business, First Impressions, which she established in 1989, has taken her across the United States, developing and presenting workshops for professional organizations and corporations on professional appearance, nonverbal communication, business etiquette and presentation skills. A trainer of new consultants for an international image firm, Beauty for All Seasons, and an award-winning consultant herself, Nancy has another book to her credit: *The New Professional Image from Business Casual to the Boardroom.*

Her career experience includes being national education director for Baby Lock sergers and sewing machines. She also managed a retail fabric store whose volume doubled under her direction. Nancy now appears regularly as a guest sewing expert on QVC national shopping network and has produced nine instructional sewing videos. She also contributes frequently to sewing publications such as McCall's Patterns magazine, Sew News and Update Newsletters.

Her education includes a degree in accounting with a minor in fashion merchandising and a master's degree in corporate communications. Nancy also is trained and certified with the Professional Image Institute, Beauty for All Seasons, Karla Jordan, Doncaster and Palmer/Pletsch—all fashion- and image-oriented companies.

She has chaired the fashion department advisory council for William Woods College, and has taught personal development courses for a prominent international training company.

Nancy and her husband, Richard, who also runs a home-based business, have five children. They live in St. Louis, Missouri.

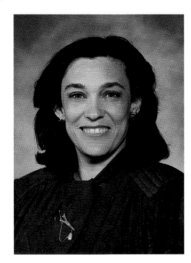

Nancy's own image-improvement evolution through the '80s inspired her to share her new-found strategies with others in the '90s.

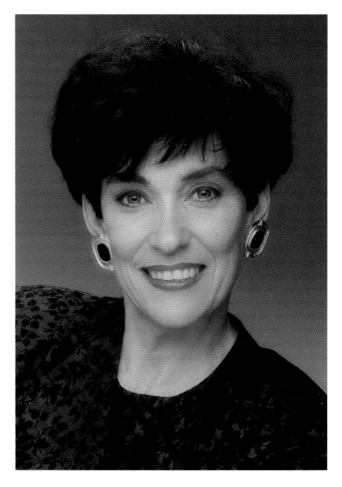

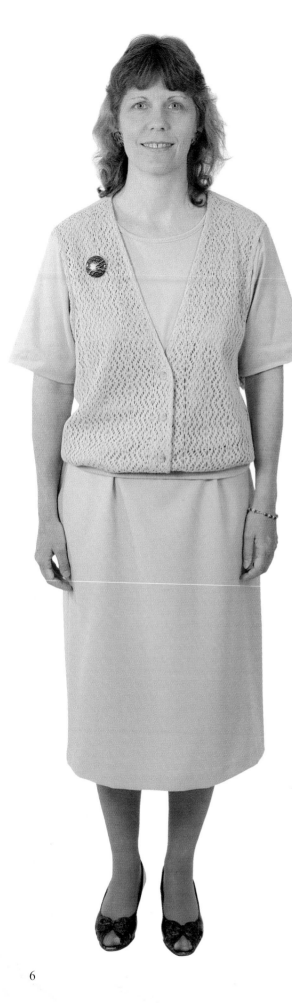

Who
appears more
confident?

◆

Who looks
more
polished?

◆

Which woman
would you
hire for a
management
position?

◆

Who is more
influential
in the
community?

◆

Who looks
more physically
fit?

Why Bother Looking Good...
The Importance of Image

Your Mom—bless her heart—loves you for who you are on the inside. But let's face it. The rest of the world judges you—and me too—based in large part on what they see on the outside.

Studies show that in just the first 15 seconds, a new person meeting you forms more than a dozen surprisingly profound impressions about you and your life, based almost entirely on your appearance.

Consider the two women in the photographs at left.

Guess What?

Both photos are the same woman! But the differences in her appearance cause most people to make vastly different assumptions about the "two" women.

Now—

Let's set aside the reactions of other people. There is another compelling reason for looking our best: our OWN reaction to ourselves.

The average American woman is said to see her reflection 55 times DAILY. That means 55 opportunities to react "Ah, YES" or "Oh, NO!" to her own appearance. What a confidence builder...or confidence destroyer...that can be.

All of this is exciting news, because those impressions—others' and our own—are under our control. By looking the way we'd like to be perceived, we can magically cause others to see us that way. And in many cases, their perception soon becomes our reality.

But if appearances are so important, why doesn't everyone look wonderful every day?

Women consistently list three reasons for looking less than their best:

1.   Not enough money

2.   Not enough time

3.   Don't know how

The GOOD NEWS is that with the know-how you are about to gain, you can look your personal best even in a hurry and on a shoestring budget if necessary. The first element of that vital "know-how" is knowing all about yourself—the exciting adventure of analyzing YOU.

CHAPTER 1

Getting to Know You

Looking wonderful is less about fashion—designers dictating what's "in" and what's "out"—than about function—what works best for YOU. Your unique sense of style will begin to unfold as you explore:

♦ **Personal Style** - Who you are and what age you want to project.

♦ **Lifestyle** - What you do and what clothing you need for those activities.

♦ **Color Style** - The colors that bring out your best features and enhance your personal coloring.

♦ **Body Style** - What challenge areas do you want to camouflage; what assets can you spotlight?

♦ **Clothes Style** - What styles create the visual illusion of a perfectly proportioned you?

Personal Style

Have you ever owned an outfit that, every time you wore it, gave you the wonderful feeling of "This is just ME"?

It undoubtedly was a reflection of your personal style—your inborn tendency to feel the most authentic in a particular way of putting yourself together.

Use the following quiz to help define the various elements of YOUR personal style. In each category, circle the choice you find most comfortable. Then total your answers by letter.

♦ The choices should relate to your lifestyle, but not be dictated by it. If your reality is life with toddlers and most mornings you live in a sweatshirt with baby food on the shoulder... select the looks you'd *like* to be wearing. You work in a bank and wear rigid navy blue suits, but long for more flair? Select the styles you'd choose in a less restrictive situation.

♦ This quiz focuses on your **feelings** about your look. There's plenty of time to address those important lifestyle considerations later.

The pages that follow this quiz describe four personal style categories. You may find yourself primarily in one of the descriptions, or discover that you are a combination. You may even vary depending on your mood. Your goal is to determine what wardrobe support the person you really are!

Personal Style Quiz

You want others to perceive you as:
A. *Gracious, refined, well-mannered*
B. *Friendly, informal, perky*
C. *Sophisticated, self-assured, exciting*
D. *Soft, feminine, charming*

Which statement describes your clothing tastes?
A. *Tailored, understated elegance*
B. *Simple, casual, comfortable*
C. *Fashion-forward, creative*
D. *Soft, sensual, graceful*

Which best describes your makeup look?
A. *Subtle and sophisticated; clear colors and polished application*
B. *Minimal makeup, natural, healthy glow*
C. *The newest, boldest colors and applications*
D. *Soft or frosted pastel colors; delicate look*

Which clothing shapes do you prefer?
A. *Tailored, symmetrical, sleek*
B. *Simple, easy, sporty lines*
C. *Bold, asymmetrical, angular*
D. *Soft and flowing*

Your idea of a great evening out is:
A. *A symphony concert*
B. *A barbeque with friends*
C. *An avant-garde theater production*
D. *A candlelight dinner for two*

If you were taking dancing lessons, they would be:
A. *Ballroom*   C. *Jazz*
B. *Country line dancing*   D. *Ballet*

Which group of women do you identify with in fashion terms?
A. *Nancy Reagan, Jackie Onassis, Diane Sawyer*
B. *Sally Field, Christie Brinkley, Jane Fonda*
C. *Cher, Diana Ross, Bianca Jagger*
D. *Elizabeth Taylor, Jane Seymour, Jaclyn Smith*

Besides solids, which patterns and textures dominate your wardrobe?

A.
Tailored stripes & plaids, paisleys

B.
Tweeds, corduroys, herring-bones

C.
Bold geometrics and splashy florals

D.
Soft florals, sheers and laces

Assuming your hair would cooper-ate, which hairstyle would you wear?

A.
Neat, smooth and simple

B.
Short and tousled

C.
Sleek and asymmetri-cal

D.
Softly curled and feathered

You'd most likely accessorize your hair with:

A. *Sleek combs or a Chanel bow*

B. *Simple headband or ponytail clip*

C. *A stunning hat*

D. *Lace bow or flowers*

Which shoe would you select with casual clothes?

A. *Spectator pumps*

B. *Loafers*

C. *Low-heeled boots*

D. *Ballet flats*

With dressier clothes you probably wear:

A. *Plain or spectator mid-heel pumps*

B. *Low-heel pumps*

C. *Multicolor high heels*

D. *Bow-trimmed flats*

Which statement describes your accessories?

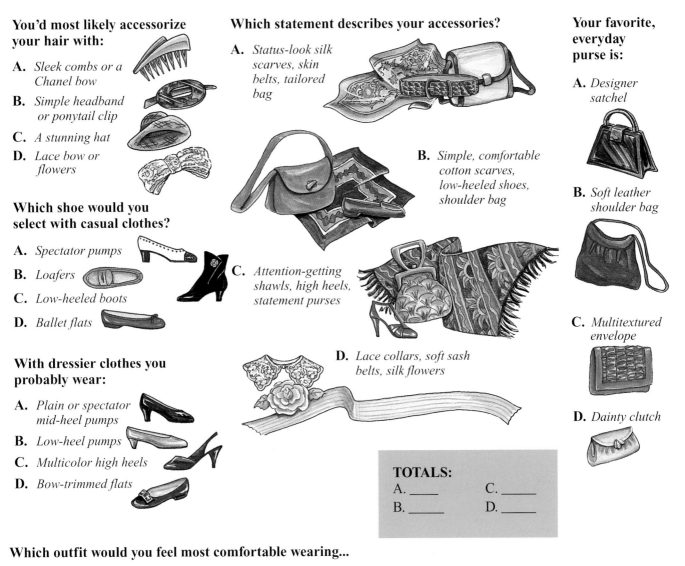

A. *Status-look silk scarves, skin belts, tailored bag*

B. *Simple, comfortable cotton scarves, low-heeled shoes, shoulder bag*

C. *Attention-getting shawls, high heels, statement purses*

D. *Lace collars, soft sash belts, silk flowers*

Your favorite, everyday purse is:

A. *Designer satchel*

B. *Soft leather shoulder bag*

C. *Multitextured envelope*

D. *Dainty clutch*

TOTALS:
A. _____   C. _____
B. _____   D. _____

Which outfit would you feel most comfortable wearing...

For a casual Saturday outing?

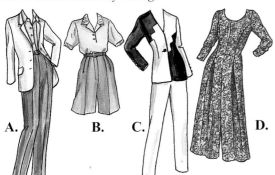

A.   **B.**   **C.**   **D.**

For a luncheon?

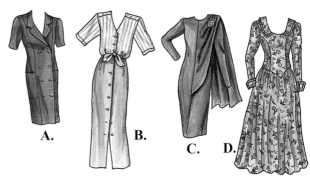

A.   **B.**   **C.**   **D.**

For a special party?

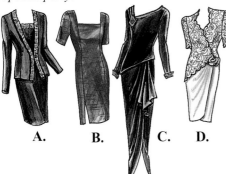

A.   **B.**   **C.**   **D.**

For a business meeting?

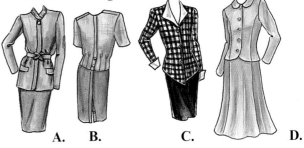

A.   **B.**   **C.**   **D.**

9

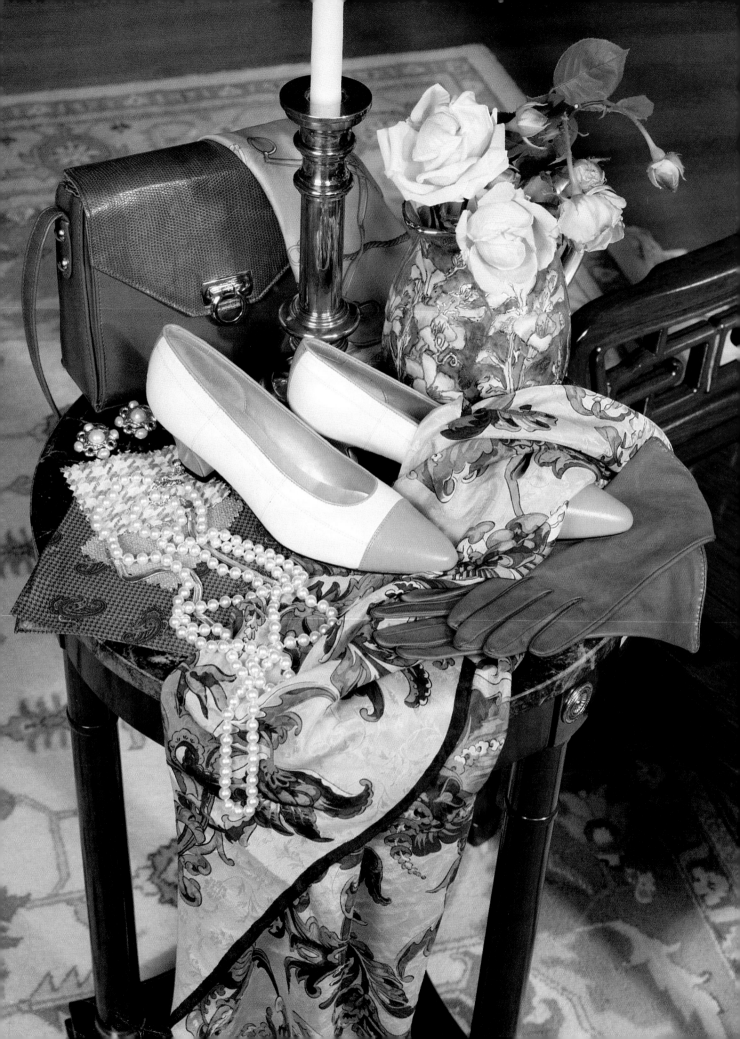

Tailored Classic

If more of your answers are "A," you are probably a Tailored Classic. This is the base point from which other personal styles are defined.

The Tailored Classic prefers an understated, refined and elegant look. She forgoes the latest fad in favor of a more timeless style every time.

Balance and symmetry characterize her clothing lines.

FABRICS: She usually chooses a solid color or small pattern like herringbone or houndstooth. In prints, her preferences run toward soft florals or controlled geometrics. She avoids fabrics that are very bulky or very clingy, opting instead for fine woolens, silkies, jersey.

EVENING: Her evening look is more likely to be velvet or satin rather than glitzy metallic.

ACCESSORIES: Her jewelry choices are usually softly rounded and symmetrical, in elegant materials like pearls and semi-precious stones. Classic pumps and two-color spectator styles make up the bulk of her shoe wardrobe. Her purse or briefcase is structured rather than soft.

HAIR: Her hairstyle is generally soft and sleek, with a definite style and "on purpose" look.

MAKEUP: She typically chooses conservative makeup colors and applies them with a polished plan, rather than picking up the season's newest color in shadow or lipstick.

WARNING: The Tailored Classic woman can avoid fashion extremes until she ends up with a look that is too safe and conservative—even BORING. She may need to enliven her look with a few interesting fashion touches.

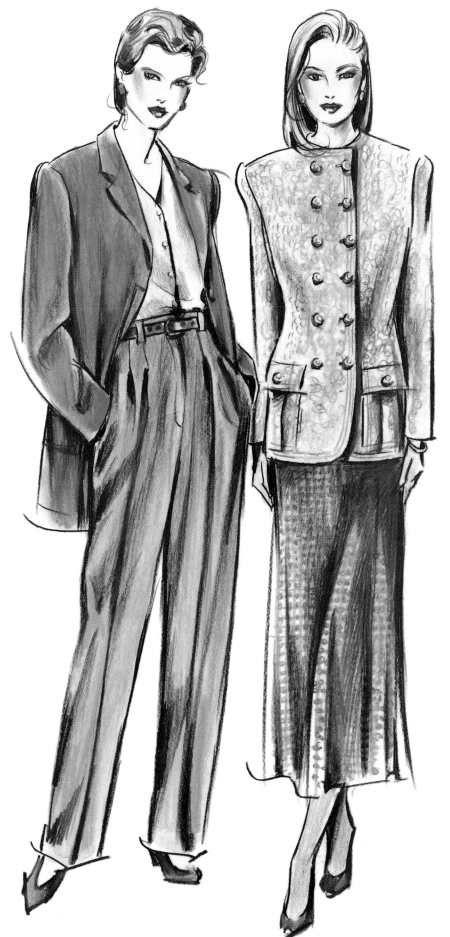

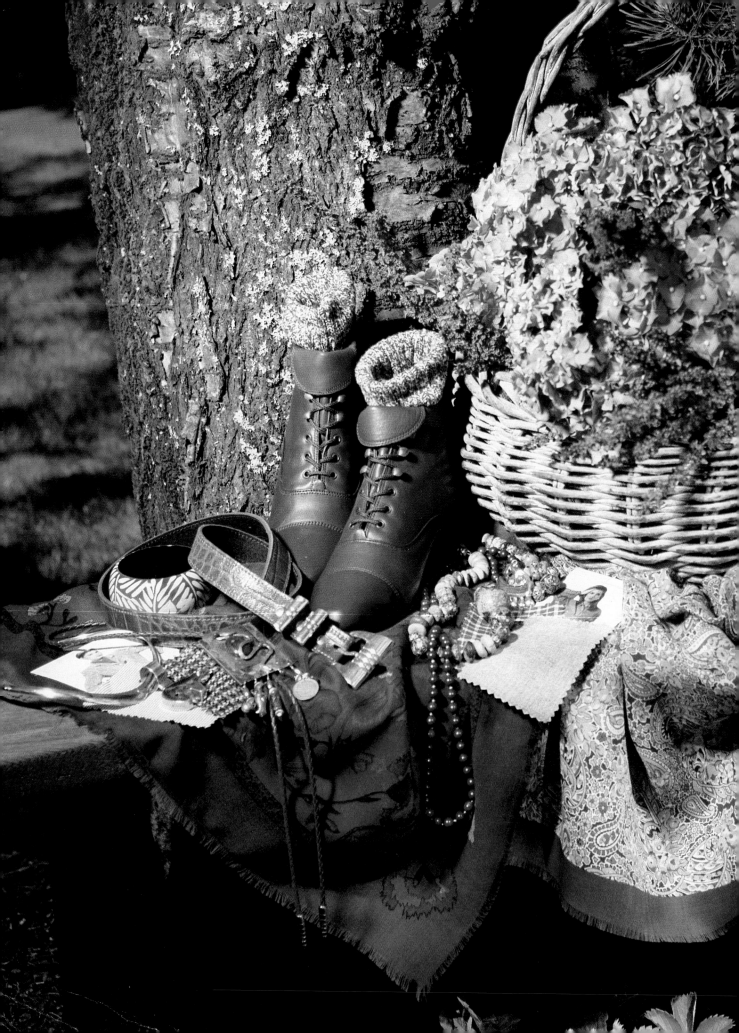

Sporty Natural

If you answered mostly B, you are a Sporty Natural, the typical "girl next door," a very easy-going, casual person who is not willing to suffer for the sake of fashion. Comfort is a basic requirement for your wardrobe choices.

FABRICS: A Sporty Natural leans toward durable fabrics like denim and corduroy, shirting plaids and stripes, tweeds and textured hand-knits.

EVENING: She chooses a relaxed look, even for dressy occasions: pants and a dressy sweater or perhaps a long plaid skirt and soft blouse.

ACCESSORIES: Her jewelry is basic, perhaps a gold chain and little stud earrings or maybe natural wood pieces. She chooses loafers or sneakers for casual wear and low-heeled pumps for dress. She probably carries a soft shoulder bag.

HAIR: A tousled, easy-care hairstyle is the Sporty Natural's trademark.

MAKEUP: Her makeup is minimal—perhaps just blush and lip color.

WARNING: A sporty Natural can easily look "under-dressed." She needs a precision haircut, careful makeup choices and a few more polished accessories to avoid looking sloppy.

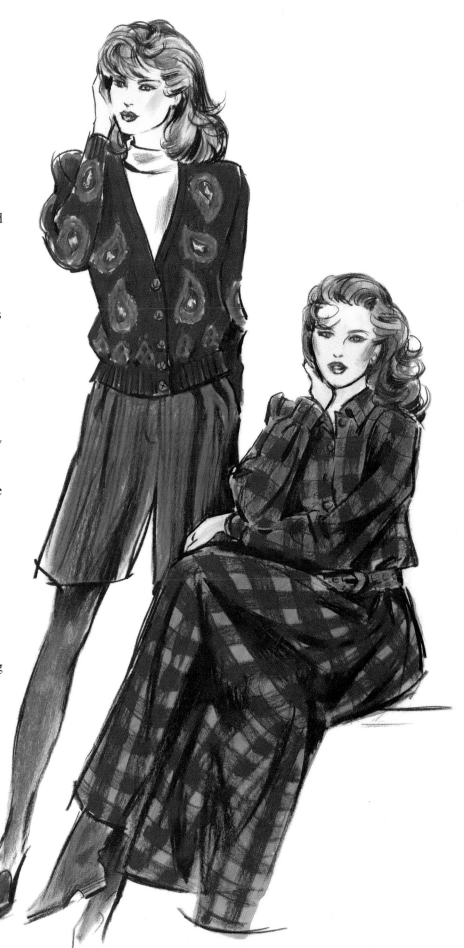

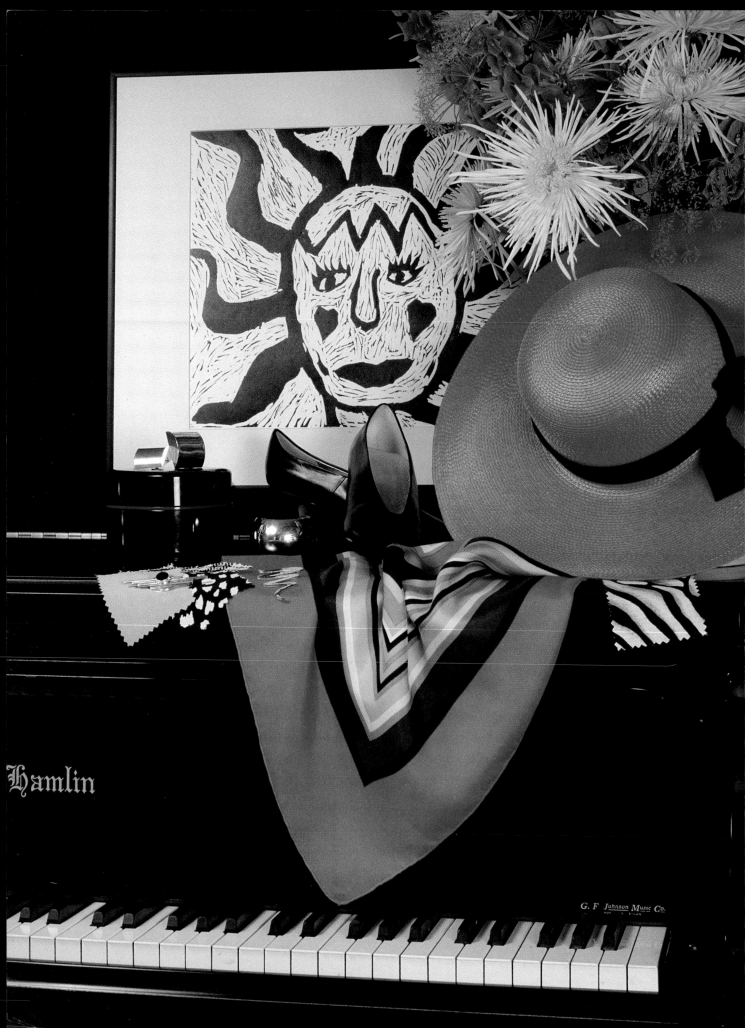

High-Fashion Dramatic

Mostly C answers make you a High-Fashion Dramatic. The legendary "clotheshorse," you love to be seen in the latest styles, and comfort factors take a back seat to fashion. Angular or asymmetrical designs are among your favorites. Yours is a striking, head-turning look.

FABRICS: Solid colors—often brightly contrasting ones—and plain weaves like gabardine, crepe and jersey fill a Dramatic's closet. Her print choices are usually bold, over-sized geometrics or abstracts.

EVENING: A Dramatic typically dresses up in all-out glitz and glamour. Metallics and jewels decorate her body-conscious silhouettes.

ACCESSORIES: Her jewelry pieces make a bold statement, maybe large geometric pieces in shiny metals, or perhaps one-of-a-kind wearable art items. Her purse is oversized and makes a statement in texture or style. She has a whole wardrobe of brightly colored shoes and boots.

HAIR: Her hairstyle is likely to be very sleek and short or very long and flamboyant.

MAKEUP: The latest application techniques and the boldest colors are a Dramatic's makeup preference.

WARNING: A High-Fashion Dramatic's look can easily become overdone and can intimidate her less fashion-forward friends. She may need to consciously tone down her look, especially in a corporate environment.

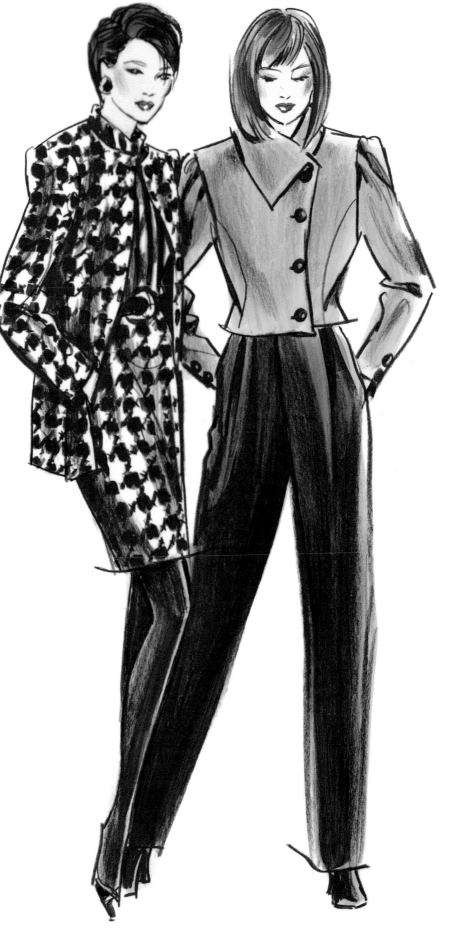

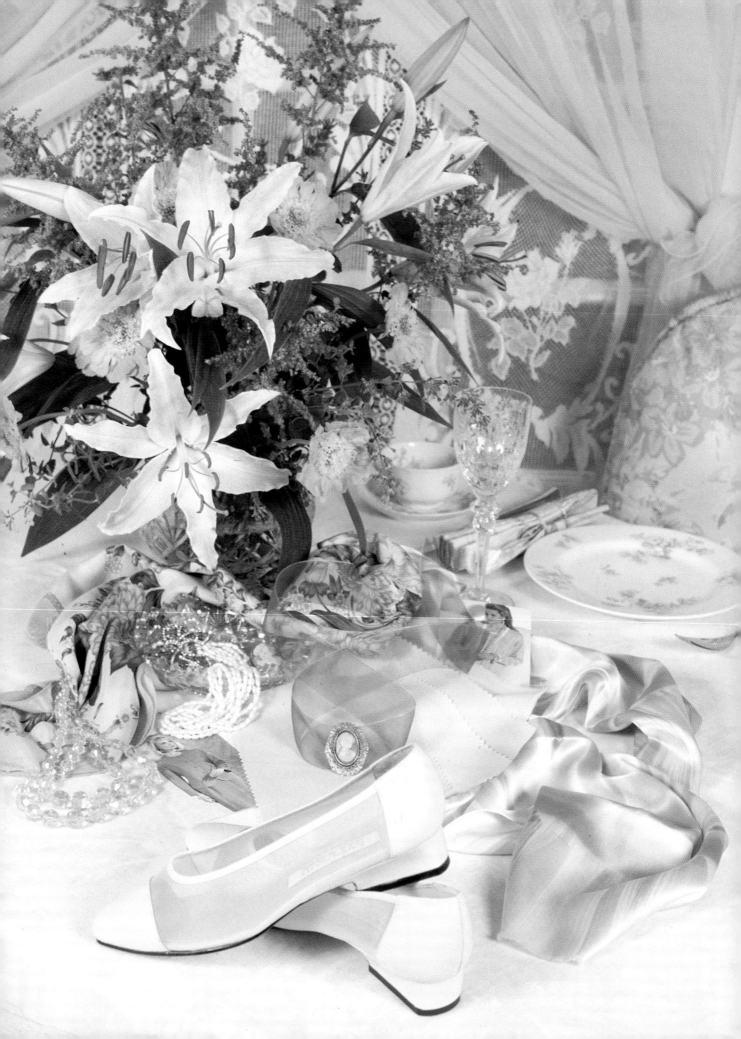

Feminine Romantic

The Feminine Romantic answers mostly D. She has a delicate, soft appearance and consistently prefers soft, flowing silhouettes, soft colors and rounded detailing like scallops and ruffles.

FABRICS: Her fabric preferences are lightweight and drapable. Soft jerseys, silks, sheer voile and soft cottons top her list. In prints she is likely to select pastel florals. Lace collars and other lace accents are popular.

EVENING: Her formalwear choices tend toward the softness of velvet and chiffon or the romance of lace.

ACCESSORIES: Femininity is the key to accessory choices for the Romantic. Her jewelry box is probably full of pearls, bow motifs, cameos and antique-look pieces. Her shoes are light and airy, with narrow straps, or perhaps bow-trimmed flats. Her handbag is small and soft.

HAIR: A soft, full style with curls or waves can be long or short. Bows, barrettes and headbands are popular with Romantics.

MAKEUP: The Romantic is likely to choose very soft pinky or peachy shades and apply them with a light touch.

WARNING: The Feminine Romantic needs to be careful to avoid appearing "little-girlish," especially in business situations.

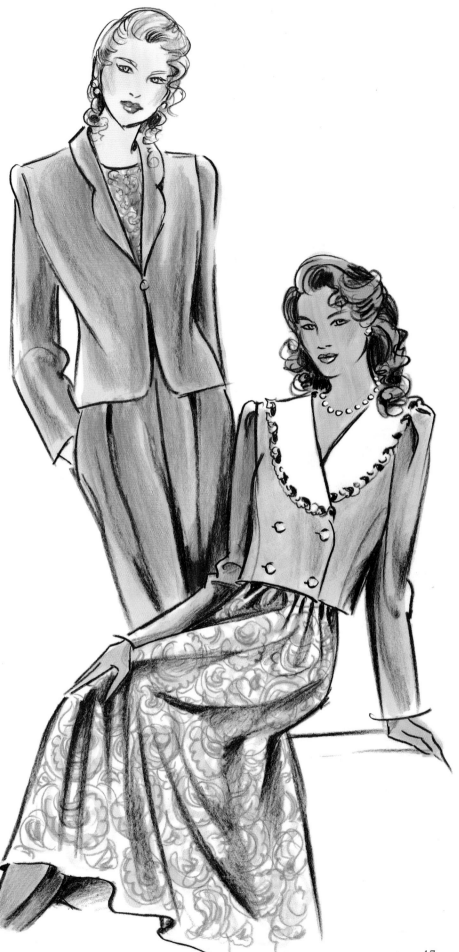

Understand YOUR Personal Style

You may be Tailored Classic, or Sporty Natural, or High-Fashion Dramatic, or Feminine Romantic. Or you may see elements of yourself in more than one of these categories. You may be one of the four described here, but do everything with flair, adding colorful, ethnic or one-of-a-kind items to your wardrobe. That could mean you are a Creative Romantic, or some other unique category.

The purpose of defining Personal Style is not to force you into a particular cubbyhole, but to help you identify the various elements of a look that are consistently comfortable for you. When you select major wardrobe pieces in your predominant style category, you'll have a more consistent look and a more flexible wardrobe.

Understanding your personal style can also help you avoid costly buying mistakes. You won't be a slave to fashion or impulse buying. I vividly remember the Christmas when I sewed beautiful Victorian dresses for my twin daughters... then went out and bought yards of fabric to make a matching dress for myself. As I was preparing to stay up all night sewing, it dawned on me that the style was incompatible with my own Tailored Classic taste. I put the fabric in the attic (for their Christmas dresses some future year) and went to bed.

Lifestyle

What do you DO all day? What occasions do you need to dress for?

Those "Lifestyle" factors are an important consideration in planning a wardrobe that works. This is an area that may need frequent reassessment as your life evolves. Student...young single professional...working parent...at-home mom... returning professional... retiree. All of our lives are a succession of roles.

We often wear a variety of hats during a single stage! It's important to build a wardrobe that meets ALL our needs.

♦ Many career women have a closet full of wonderful suits, but dress like a "ragbag" in their leisure hours.

♦ At-home moms often have a wide variety of casual clothes, but "nothing to wear" for a special occasion.

Take a look at your lifestyle, using the chart. Use your finished chart to determine the percentage of total time you spend in each category of activities, then create a pie graph to give you a visual picture of your wardrobe needs.

Lifestyle Chart

	HOURS SPENT DAILY							Weekly Total
	Sun.	Mon.	Tues.	Wed.	Thur.	Fri.	Sat.	
Professional Time								
Full-time work								
Part-time work								
Volunteer work								
Family Time								
Mothering								
Cooking								
Shopping								
Other household activities								
_____								
_____								
Social Time								
Church								
Entertaining								
Entertainment (dining out, cultural activities)								
Recreation Time								
Sewing								
Arts/Crafts								
Sports								
Sleeping/relaxing								
Other _____								
_____								
_____								

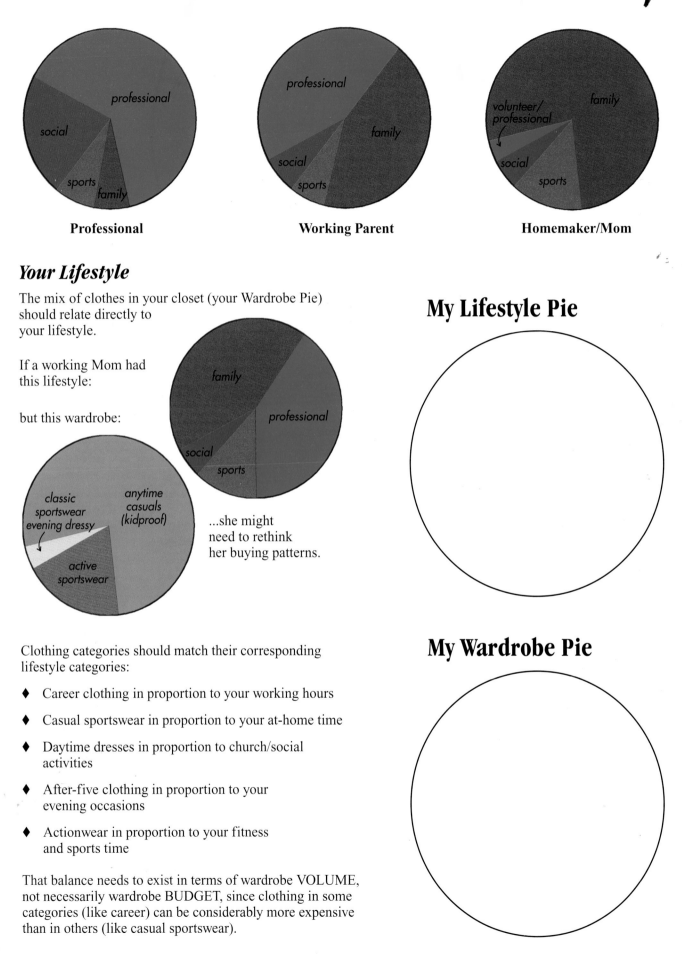

Professional   **Working Parent**   **Homemaker/Mom**

Your Lifestyle

The mix of clothes in your closet (your Wardrobe Pie) should relate directly to your lifestyle.

If a working Mom had this lifestyle:

but this wardrobe:

...she might need to rethink her buying patterns.

My Lifestyle Pie

Clothing categories should match their corresponding lifestyle categories:

♦   Career clothing in proportion to your working hours

♦   Casual sportswear in proportion to your at-home time

♦   Daytime dresses in proportion to church/social activities

♦   After-five clothing in proportion to your evening occasions

♦   Actionwear in proportion to your fitness and sports time

That balance needs to exist in terms of wardrobe VOLUME, not necessarily wardrobe BUDGET, since clothing in some categories (like career) can be considerably more expensive than in others (like casual sportswear).

My Wardrobe Pie

Career Style

Some Special Considerations

Back in the '70s, women sneaked into the workplace disguised as men. Remember the navy blue "clone suit," white shirt and red bow tie? A lot has changed since then. Women have earned their place in the corporate world and today our unique attributes are not only accepted, they're celebrated.

That acceptance brings us the flexibility to express our own style in a wide variety of professional clothing. So it's important to analyze the message you'd like your professional look to send, and dress accordingly. The range of acceptable messages varies with the type of work you do.

Businesses	Law, Banking, Finance, High-level Corporate	Insurance, Teaching, Real Estate, Sales	Advertising, Art, Fashion, Writing, Entertainment
Messages	Authoritative Conservative Competent	Trustworthy Approachable Knowledgeable	Creative Individual Contemporary
Clothes	Matched skirted suits and classic dresses in highest quality and subdued style and color	Unmatched suits, jacketed dresses, sweater jackets, tailored trousers	More flamboyant styles accepted, even expected; bold colors, unique accessories

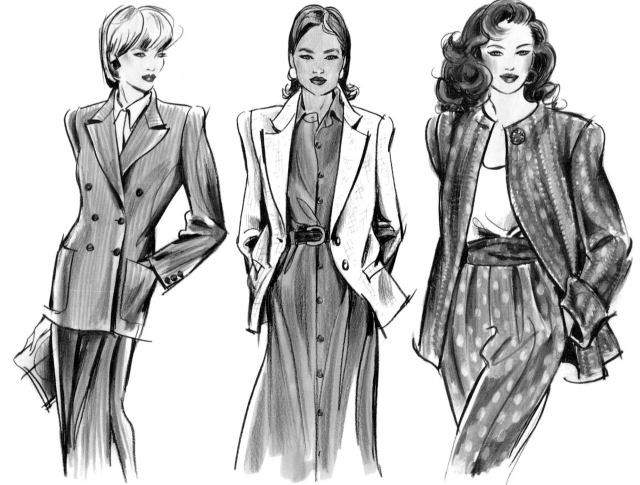

like the brown belt on the blue

If you think dressing for a conservative career has to be boring, take heart. Even a traditional navy suit can express your individuality, with accessory touches drawn from your Personal Style and colors from your seasonal color palette (page 25).

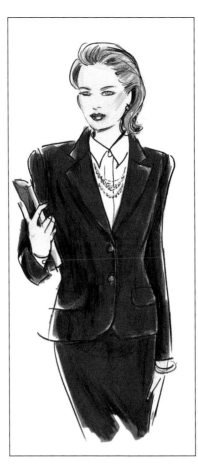

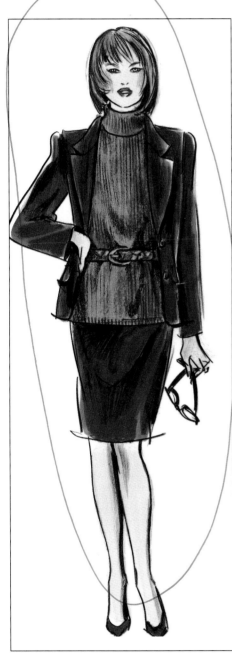

For detailed advice about business dressing at every level from business casual to the boardroom, read the book *The New Professional Image* by Susan Bixler and Nancy Nix-Rice.

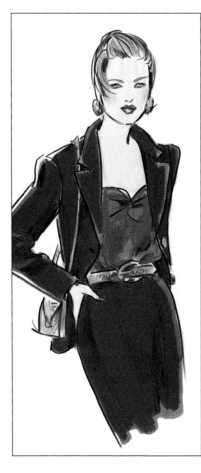

Note carefully the wardrobe choices of the women at the next higher level in your company. By dressing for the job you'd like to have, you can subtly make it easier for superiors to envision you in that role.

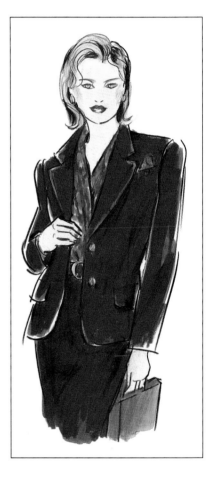

Working at Home

The growing cadre of women who work from their homes face special wardrobe challenges. Meetings with clients may require the conventional dress for their profession. But home-office time requires a polished, casual wardrobe, not a collection of sloppy sweat suits. The information on Casual Capsules in Chapter 4 addresses that need.

Color Style

Color is really a magic ingredient in an effective image. Wear the right colors and your skin glows, your eyes sparkle and your hair is full of highlights.

Wearing the wrong colors you look drained and tired. Wrong colors shadow your face and create the illusions of under-eye circles and double chins.

And the color element is FREE! It doesn't cost a cent more to buy a blouse in a color that makes you sparkle than to buy it in a color that deadens you.

A more flattering color blouse doesn't take any longer to put on in the morning either!

Knowing Your Best Colors Saves Money

♦ The average American woman has at least a $2,000 investment in her closet. Just one or two outfits that hang unworn can be a costly mistake.

♦ Knowing your best colors reduces impulse buying and makes you less likely to jump on a fad color that doesn't flatter YOU. It helps you resist the "it was such a great markdown" method of selecting colors, too.

♦ Consistently shopping in your best colors creates a harmony within your wardrobe and leads to lots of happy accidents—wardrobe items that just seem to go together without conscious planning.

Nearly everyone has heard of color analysis, but few people really understand the theory behind it.

The color wheel is a systematic representation of all the colors we see, organized according to the proportion of warm yellow pigment or cool blue pigment each color contains.

Warm or Cool Undertones?

Just as colors can be classified as warm or cool, human beings can be described as having undertones to their personal coloring that are either warm or cool, depending on the relative proportions of melanin, carotene and hemoglobin in their unique body chemistry.

Because skin, hair and eyes react to the colors around them, the first step in selecting flattering colors is to match the warmth or coolness of the colors you wear to the warmth or coolness of your personal coloring.

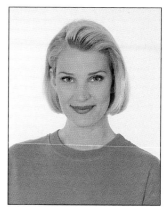

♦ Your skin, hair and eyes will **absorb** colors that match your own undertones. The result is a sparkling appearance.

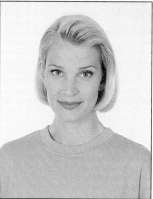

♦ But when the colors you wear are of the opposite undertone, they will be **reflected** and will deaden your appearance.

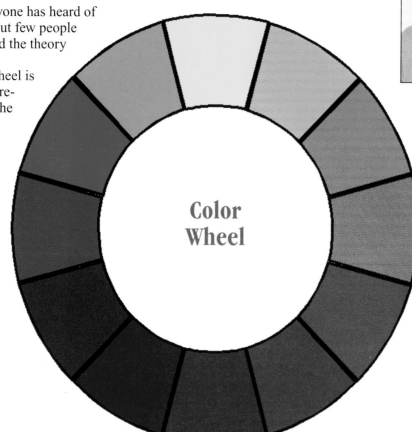

Color Wheel

Many people can determine their own undertone category—warm or cool—by holding pieces of metallic fabric near the face.

- ♦ If gold is obviously more harmonious and flattering, your undertones are probably WARM.

- ♦ If silver is noticeably more flattering, your undertones are probably COOL.

- ♦ If both metals seem equally flattering, your undertones are too subtle for this simplistic test. Read on.

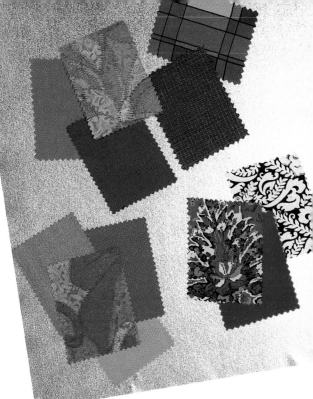

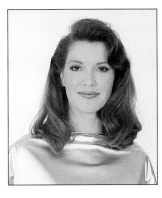 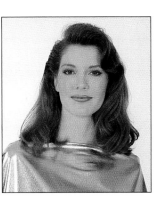

This woman has warm undertones.

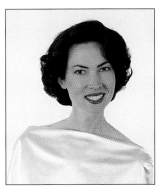 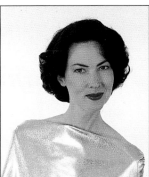

This woman has cool undertones.

Once you have determined your most enhancing metallic, simply try a sample of that metal with a color you are thinking of buying. If your metal looks right with the color, chances are the color has the right undertones for you.

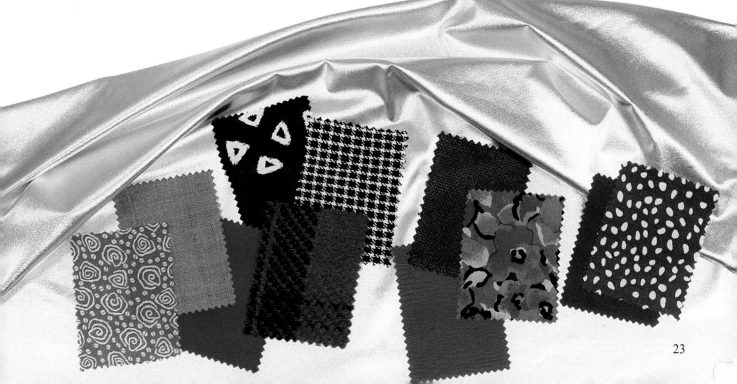

23

Color Value And Intensity

The next step in matching fashion colors to your personal coloring is the element of VALUE (the lightness or darkness of the colors you wear) and INTENSITY (pure color diminishes in intensity as increasing amounts of gray are added). Both need to relate to the softness or intensity of YOU.

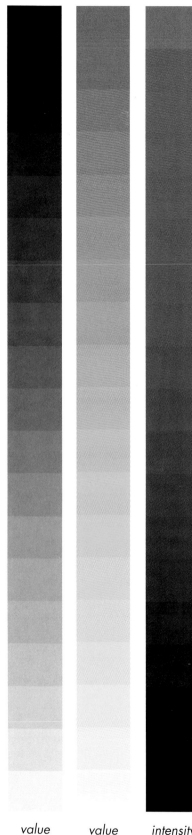

value   value   intensity

A delicate blonde could be overpowered by very intense, vivid colors.

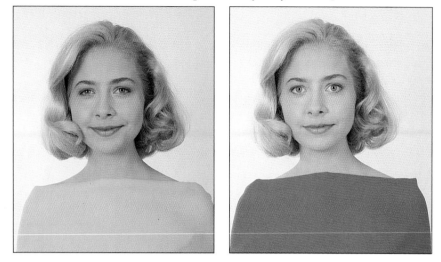

An olive-skinned brunette would look out-of-balance wearing icy pastels.

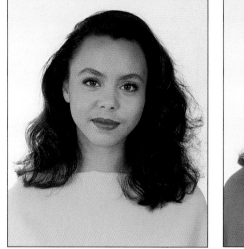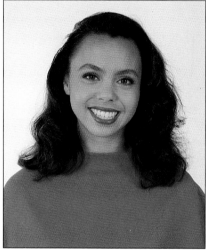

the "Four Seasons of Color"

Warm + Light = Spring	Cool + Light = Summer
Warm + Dark = Autumn	Cool + Dark = Winter

The "Four Seasons" of Color

Warm/cool and light/dark can be combined to create four categories, typically called the "Four Seasons" of color.

The four women shown here are representative of each of the "four seasons." However, dividing the whole population into only four color categories is a broad generalization. Neither the warm/cool characteristic nor the light/dark trait is really an either/or situation. There are people with varying degrees of warmth, just as there are people with many different levels of value (light/dark).

In recent years, more sophisticated color analysis systems measure both of those traits on a multistep scale. Some systems also factor in the unique skin, hair and eye colors of the individual, and define over 350 personalized color categories with specialized color recommendations for each.

For example, the green-eyed winter shown here would not wear exactly the same colors as the brown-eyed olive-skinned winter on the page at left. Even women who already know their four-season classification may want to update their color information with a newer, high-tech system.

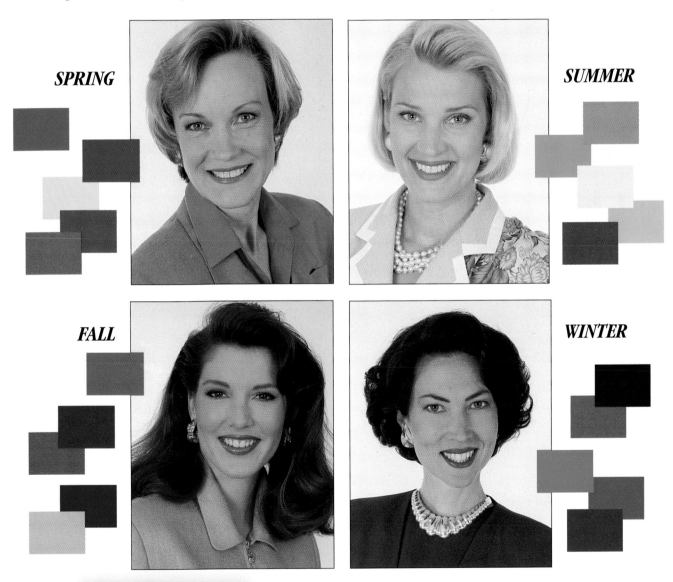

SPRING

SUMMER

FALL

WINTER

The right makeup plays an important role in looking good. Select colors that blend with your own coloring while emphasizing and enhancing it. Your color swatch palette, which is available through professional color analysis companies (see Resources, page 155), is a good guideline. For more about makeup, see Chapter 7, About Face, page 103.

Your Coloring Changes as You Age

Updating becomes particularly important as a woman ages, and skin and hair color softens. This woman was, and is, a "Summer." However, when she was younger her hair was darker and she could wear the brighter colors of a Contrasting Azure Summer*. At 45, with more and more gray in her hair, her classification changed to True Azure Summer*, and she wears softer colors.

*Beauty for All Seasons classifications.

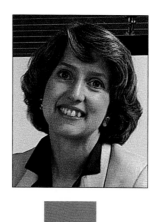
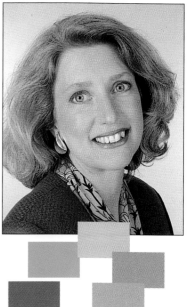

Professional Color Analysis

Color analysis is performed by a trained, professional color consultant. How do you select a top-notch consultant? After all, you will make thousands of dollars of wardrobe purchases over the years, based on her recommendations. Here are some questions to ask before you schedule an analysis:

1. **What system do you use?**
   A good consultant uses a recognized system supported by a national company, not just her own personal opinions. She should be able to explain her system in terms you understand.

2. **How were you trained?**
   Color analysis is NOT a read-the-book skill. Since it calls for making sophisticated visual comparisons, hands-on training is essential.

3. **Will we work in an individual session or a group?**
   A small group (two or three participants) can provide a good learning experience, because you can see the color impact on someone else more objectively than on yourself.

   A one-on-one analysis is obviously more personalized. A large group class or color "party" doesn't usually allow for a very sophisticated color analysis of each participant.

4. **What lighting do you use?**
   Because light affects color to a great degree, indirect natural daylight is certainly the best choice. If your analysis will take place after dark, the artificial lighting should be carefully color-corrected to simulate daylight.

5. **Do I have to take off my makeup?**
   It is impossible to do an accurate analysis with makeup on. Even though it takes a little longer, removing it is an essential step.

6. **What kind of color swatches will I receive?**
   Fabric swatches are far easier than paper samples or paint chips to match with the garments you consider buying.

   The number of swatches is important, too. Ten or 15 would be too limiting, several hundred too overwhelming. A range of 40-50 is about right for most people.

7. **What additional services are available?**
   Instruction in using your colors should be part of the basic consultation fee. Information about selecting compatible makeup colors is also important. If the colors next to your face can affect your appearance so dramatically, just imagine what the colors ON your face can do!

   Many color consultants are also qualified to help with makeup, wardrobe planning, figure analysis and personal shopping.

8. **How much does it cost?**
   As with anything else, you get what you pay for. Expect to pay from $50 to $150 or more, depending on your area. Prices vary regionally.

   A free color analysis at a home party or a department store makeup counter can be a very costly mistake, since the consultant may be more thoroughly trained to sell you her products than to offer professional color advice.

Start Wearing Your Colors

Of course your color analysis is only worth its cost if you USE it to develop your wardrobe.

Few of us can toss our entire closet and start from scratch. It can take a couple of years of conscious effort to develop a wardrobe totally keyed to your personal color palette, so be patient. Here's how to begin:

1. Resolve to make all new wardrobe purchases in your best colors.

2. Remember that the items nearest your face matter most. If you own a suit in the wrong color, add a blouse in a better shade. If a dress is the wrong color, wear a scarf in a flattering color at the neckline.

3. Don't overlook the option of dyeing an existing garment to a more flattering color.

Shop with Your Colors

1. Don't leave home without your swatch palette. You never know when a fabulous bargain might appear.

2. Compare garment colors to your swatches in daylight, since some fluorescent lighting can distort colors.

3. Understand that the colors you buy need to blend with (NOT necessarily match exactly) your color swatches.

When you shop, blend with your palette colors.

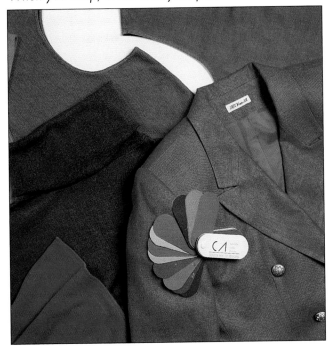

4. When considering a print or plaid, look at the item from at least 10 feet away. The dominant colors—the ones you notice most from a distance—are the ones to match to your swatches.

Sometimes colors blend to form entirely different colors when seen from a distance. Tiny prints, even in very bright colors, often look muted from a few feet away.

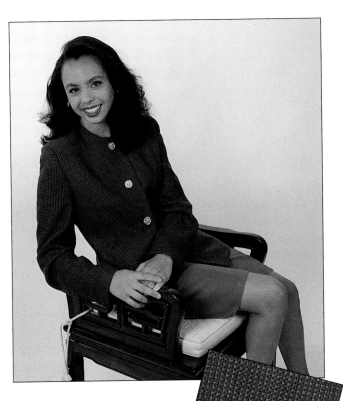

Up close, the turquoise culotte matches perfectly the turquoise in the jacket. But from a distance the two colors in the jacket visually blend, changing value to form a more muted blue that does not combine as well with the clear turquoise of the culotte.

5. When buying a color you've never worn, instead of a complete garment, which can be an expensive experiment, opt for a small, close-to-the-face item like a scarf or turtleneck. If it flatters your face, it flatters *you.*

6. Make sure you have your name and address on your swatch palette. Your colors can be expensive to replace.

Neutrals - The Building Blocks

These versatile colors provide maximum fashion mileage because they can be worn over and over without being remembered. They are also the easiest to coordinate. Neutrals can be warm or cool. Use the ones with the same undertones as your own coloring.

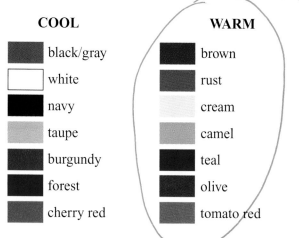

COOL	WARM
black/gray	brown
white	rust
navy	cream
taupe	camel
burgundy	teal
forest	olive
cherry red	tomato red

Select top-quality basic pieces like jackets, skirts, trousers and fine blouses in your neutrals. They will provide the building blocks for a versatile wardrobe.

Combining Neutrals

Dressing in head-to-toe neutrals can be a sophisticated, elegant look if you avoid monotony by using two of the following:

♦ Contrasts in light and dark values
♦ Interesting texture (tweed, mohair, brocade, etc.)
♦ Interesting print or fabric design
♦ Unusual or dramatic design lines

What About White?

Few people can wear bright white effectively. Creamy or softly grayed whites are often more flattering. Choose an all-white outfit only if you have lots of contrast in your own coloring (dark hair and pale skin, for example). White attracts attention, so use it to spotlight an area you'd like people to notice. It will simultaneously distract the eye from a color or style element that is not so good for you.

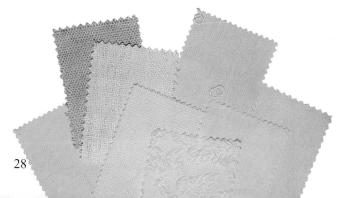

Eye Color

The composite color of your eyes is one of your most effective wardrobe colors. Worn near your face, it causes people to focus on your eyes—a big plus in any one-on-one communication situation.

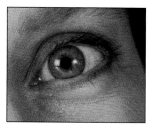

Red

Once considered purely a social-occasion color, red is today a mainstay in many women's career wardrobes as well. Everyone can wear red. If you have warm coloring, wear reds tinged with orange; if your skin tone is cool, select blue-based cherry reds.

Skin-Emphasizer Colors

Colors that fall opposite one another on the color wheel (called complementary colors) brighten or enliven one another (see page 30).

All skin tones come from the orange or red area of the color wheel. The opposite range of blue-greens are their complement.

These colors can stand alone or add a spark of excitement to a neutral outfit. Wear them when you want to attract attention, not when you'd rather blend into the crowd.

Advancing/Receding Colors

Use color to create your best illusion:

♦ **Light colors advance** and can be used to increase apparent body size.

♦ **Dark colors recede** and can be used to decrease apparent body size.

♦ **Bright and warm colors advance** and are most easily seen. Use them to emphasize or increase body areas.

♦ **Dull and cool colors recede** and are less visible. Use them to camouflage or de-emphasize body areas.

Combining Colors

Work with your color swatches to find exciting new color combinations. Here are some guidelines to get you started.

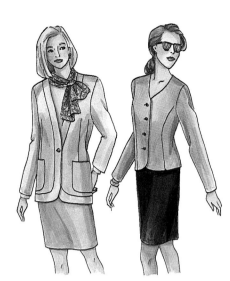

1. In a multiple-color ensemble, choose

   ♦ a major amount of one color (the suit, for example)

   ♦ a secondary amount of another color (blouse)

   ♦ just a dash of a third accent color (scarf)

Equal amounts of several colors can create an awkward appearance. In this example, a scarf, jewelry or blouse that picks up the skirt color would help balance the ensemble.

2. The easiest color schemes are:

   ♦ neutrals head to toe

   ♦ neutrals with a single color accent (blouse or accessories)

   ♦ monochromatic - light and dark versions of one color

   ♦ a multicolor print or plaid, worn with any one of its component colors

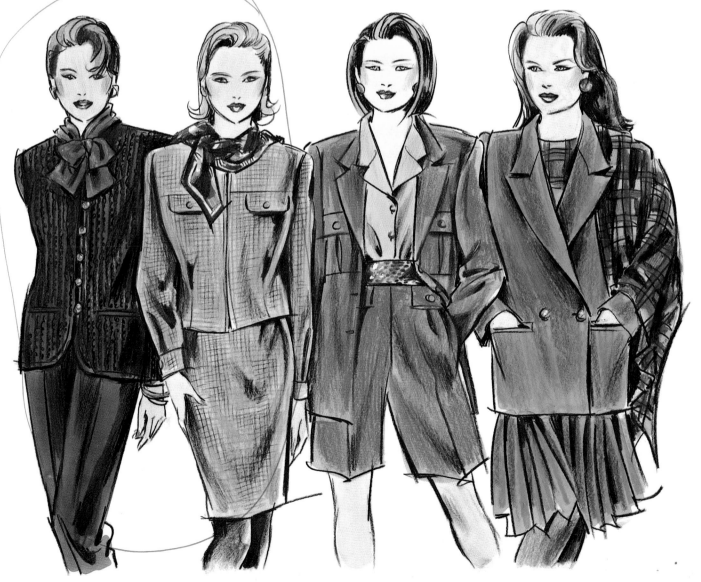

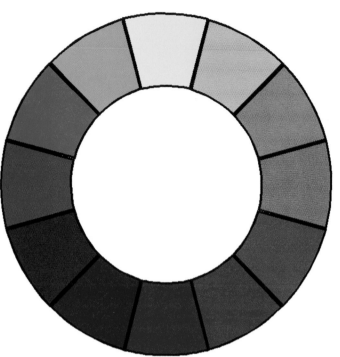

More Combinations

The color wheel can suggest more interesting color combinations for the wardrobe adventurer.

♦ **Primary colors**—red, yellow, blue—are used to make all the other colors on the color wheel.

♦ **Secondary colors**—orange, green, violet—are mixtures of two primary colors.

♦ **Tertiary colors**—red-orange, yellow-orange, yellow-green, blue-green, blue-violet, red-violet—are mixtures of one primary and one secondary color.

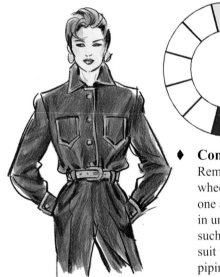

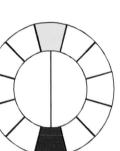

♦ **Complementary** - Remember that color wheel opposites enliven one another. Use them in unequal amounts, such as a purple jumpsuit with golden-yellow piping.

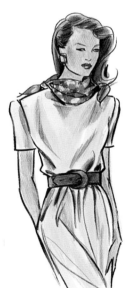

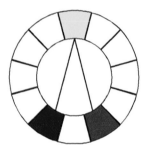

♦ **Split-complementary** - The colors on both sides of a color complement are its split-complements. Accent a yellow dress with red-violet or blue-violet, for example.

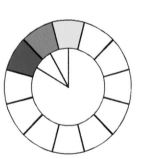

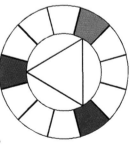

♦ **Analogous** - The colors on both sides of a color are its analogous (related) colors. If you choose blue-green, its analogous colors are blue and blue-violet to the right and green and yellow-green to the left.

A green suit with a yellow blouse and a yellow-green silk flower on the lapel would be an analogous color scheme.

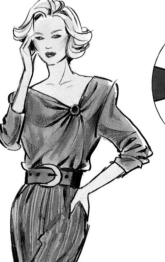

Triadic - These are the colors linked by a triangle on the color wheel. They are the most challenging to combine, but the most striking when done well.

Body Style

A recent Glamour magazine survey confirms it: Over 95 percent of American women are dissatisfied with some element of their body proportions.

That often-unjustified dissatisfaction makes it hard for women to objectively evaluate their silhouettes and select garment styles that will be flattering.

Make a Body Graph

One easy way to analyze your figure and see yourself as others see you is to make a body graph. Allow about a half hour and enlist a trusted friend to help.

1. Cut newsprint or butcher paper wider and taller than you are. (You can tape two widths together if the paper is too narrow.) Fold it in half lengthwise. Use a pen and yardstick to mark the fold line.

2. Tape the paper to a wall. Cut or crease the paper even with an uncarpeted floor.

3. Wear nonbinding underwear and no shoes. Tie elastic around your waist and wear a chain necklace to mark the base of your neck.

4. Stand with your back against the paper in normal posture, centering your body along the fold line. Look straight ahead. **Do not look up or down!**

5. Have a friend plot the points shown on the diagram below, using a pencil and non-flexing yardstick. Have them keep the yardstick close to your body and hold the opposite end so they see that it is perpendicular to the wall. They will mark the paper at the edge of yardstick next to body.

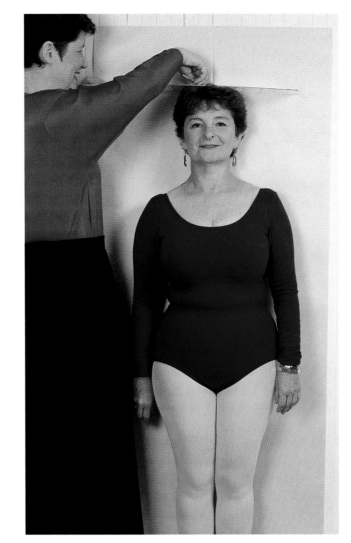

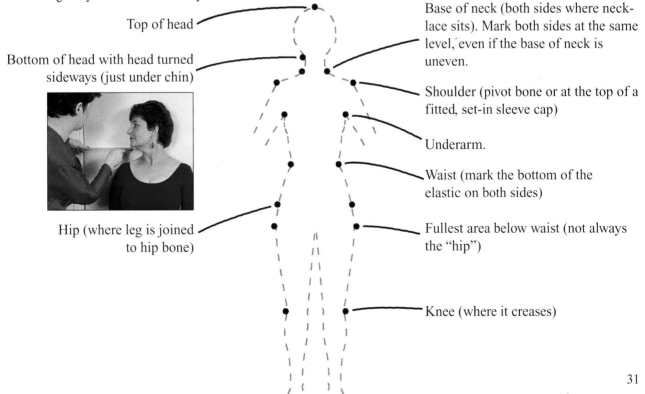

Top of head

Bottom of head with head turned sideways (just under chin)

Hip (where leg is joined to hip bone)

Base of neck (both sides where necklace sits). Mark both sides at the same level, even if the base of neck is uneven.

Shoulder (pivot bone or at the top of a fitted, set-in sleeve cap)

Underarm.

Waist (mark the bottom of the elastic on both sides)

Fullest area below waist (not always the "hip")

Knee (where it creases)

6. Step away and, with paper still taped to wall, fold the paper in half, matching the bottom of your feet with the top of your head. Fold it in half again and once again, creasing it into eight sections.

NOTE: The "perfectly" proportioned figure is eight heads tall. That is, the total height of the body is eight times the measurement of the head, divided as shown on the following page.

7. Step back against paper and have friend trace your silhouette, connecting the dots to create your shape. For accuracy, pencil must be perpendicular to wall.

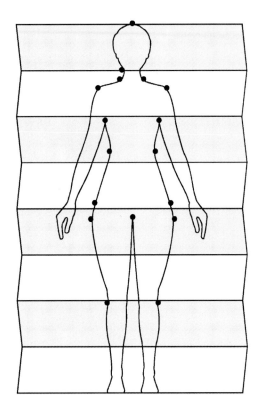

8. Draw a line straight out from the base of the neck in both directions to above the shoulder dots, parallel to the nearest fold line.

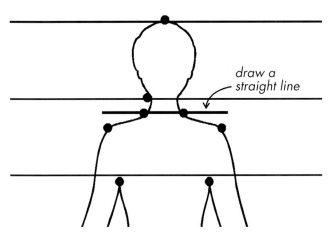

draw a straight line

9. Draw a dotted line box that connects your shoulder dots to fullest hip area dots.

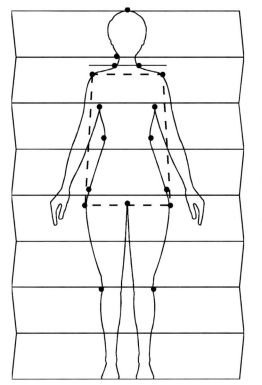

Fullest area may be low in thigh area.

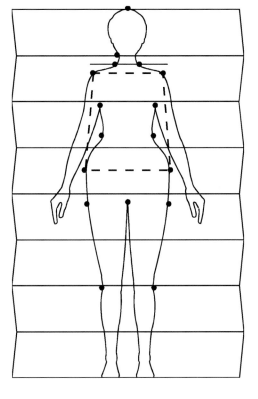

-or it may be just below the waist.

Excerpted from the upcoming Palmer/Pletsch book, **Fit for Real People**.

Your graph doesn't look much like Barbie? No surprise! The average American woman is under 5'4" and weighs about 145 pounds. To even approach the impossibly perfect Barbie-doll silhouette, she would have to lose 7" in the waist, gain 12" in the bust, be 6' tall and have 4"-long feet.

The true measure of confidence is a woman who understands her own body and dresses as if she's proud of it! So compare yourself to the more realistic "perfect" proportions at right only to identify your personal figure challenges and—equally important—your figure assets.

The asset part is critical. We can readily spot our own faults... and imagine additional ones we don't really have. But the only way to successfully camouflage those areas is by calling attention to other areas—the assets.

Now Compare Yourself to "Perfect" Proportions

"Ideal" Proportions:

Shoulders slope 1¾" from neck base for a size 10; up to 2" for a size 20.

Underarm is halfway between top of head and hip

Waist is halfway between underarm and hip

Hip divides body in half

Hips are 1" narrower than shoulders for garments to fall freely over hips

Knee is halfway between hip and feet

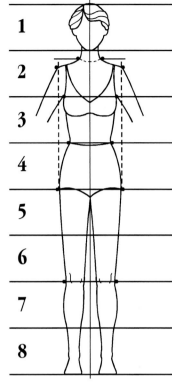

If your...

Shoulders slope ½" more or less than the ideal, you are sloping or square.

Waist is more than 1" above or below the ideal, you are short- or long-waisted.

Leg length is more than 1" longer or shorter than half your body length, you are long- or short-legged.

Use the information above as you fill out the Body Style Worksheet on the next page.

Now examine the box around your torso. If you have...

Balanced hip and shoulder width, defined waist	Shoulders narrower than hips	Shoulders wider than hips	Balanced hip and shoulder, no defined waist
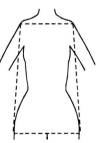		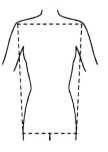	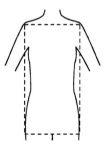

Your silhouette is...

Hourglass	Triangle	Inverted Triangle	Rectangle
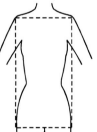	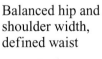		

Record your observations on the chart. Your basic bone structure is a genetic gift. It won't change with diet or exercise. The good news is that each silhouette type can look evenly proportioned with flattering wardrobe choices. For guidance, see page 35-53, and especially the chart on page 36.

Your Body Style Worksheet

Body Size

Height _____ Short (under 5'3") _____ Average (5'3"- 5'6") _____ Tall (over 5'6")

Weight _____ Slender _____ Average _____ Heavy

Body Shape (Silhouette — Use Body Graph)

Measure shoulder width (_____"), waist (_____") and hip (_____"). Circle your predominant silhouette below:

Hourglass   Triangle   Inverted Triangle   Rectangle

Note: The triangle and inverted triangle woman with a defined waist has that advantage of the hourglass figure—take advantage of it!

Body Proportions (Use Body Graph and compare to "Perfect Proportions" on page 33.)

Head Size _____ Small _____ Average _____ Large (Average head fits between first two lines.)

Shoulders (For height and slope, measure from shoulder dot up to line drawn out from neck base.)

_____ Even height _____ Uneven Left lower by _____ " Right lower by _____ "

_____ Sloping _____ Average _____ Square

_____ Narrow _____ Average _____ Broad

Note: Average shoulder width (neck base to shoulder) is 4¾" in pattern size 10, up to 5½" in size 20.

Waist

_____ Small _____ Average _____ Thick

_____ Short _____ Average _____ Long

_____ Even height _____ Uneven Left lower by _____ " Right lower by _____ "

Hips

_____ Small _____ Average _____ Full

_____ Even _____ Uneven Left lower by _____ " Right lower by _____ "

Legs

_____ Short _____ Average _____ Long

UPPER LEGS: _____ Short _____ Average _____ Long

LOWER LEGS: _____ Short _____ Average _____ Long

Profile (Study your profile in the mirror.)

Bust: _____ Small _____ Average _____ Full _____ Low _____ Average _____ High

Tummy: _____ Flat _____ Average _____ Full

Derriere: _____ Flat _____ Average _____ Full

Clothes Style

Anyone, with any body type, can create the illusion of more perfectly balanced proportions through her choice of clothes. It's largely a matter of revealing assets and concealing challenge areas through optical illusion.

Five elements of design can help you achieve your figure goals:

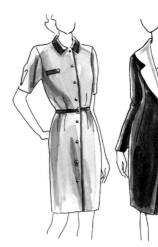

- ♦ **Scale**—design details that are proportionally smaller make the body appear larger while larger details make the body look smaller.

- ♦ **Line**—the viewer's eye follows the lines of clothing. Vertical lines draw the eye up and down, adding height and diminishing width. Horizontal lines do the opposite.

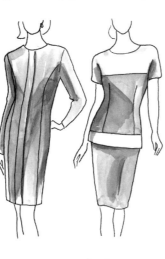

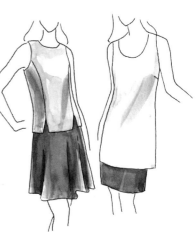

- ♦ **Proportion**—equal proportions in clothing are less flattering than unbalanced ones.

- ♦ **Color**—light, bright, warm colors attract the eye and make areas they cover appear larger. Weightier, more subdued colors diminish.

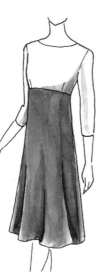

Each garment is made up of two types of lines.

Outside line is the outline or silhouette of the garment shape.

Inside lines are the details like seams, buttons, trims, pleats and lapels

- ♦ **Texture**—fuzzy, tweedy textures add visual bulk while smooth surfaces minimize. Shiny, reflective fabrics enlarge; matte surfaces diminish.

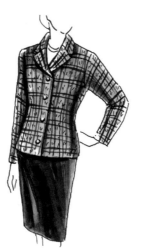

35

Outside Lines

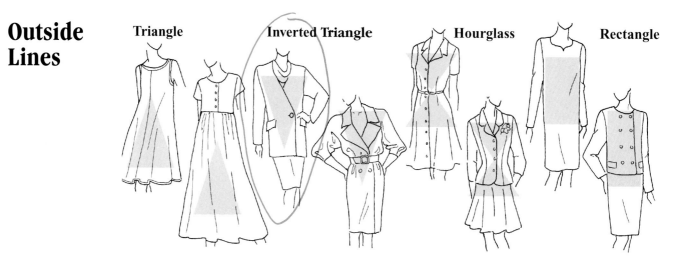

Triangle   Inverted Triangle   Hourglass   Rectangle

Most garments can be classified easily into the same four basic shapes used to classify bodies on page 33. Simply draw a mental outline around the garment. What shape did you draw?

In general, the most pleasing outside lines are those that relate to the individual's body type. They are also the easiest-to-fit styles.

♦ Inverted triangle bodies camouflage their heavy torsos when they select inverted triangle styles to emphasize their dominant shoulders and slim hips.

♦ Hourglass bodies need waistline definition in garments to emphasize their best feature.

♦ Rectangular fashions camouflage the lack of waistline definition in a rectangular body type.

♦ Triangular fashions obscure the hipline challenge area for a triangle body type.

Of course each body type can wear any of the four outside lines, but some will be more flattering than others.

If your body is...   *A garment with this outside line would...*

If your body is...				
△	be easy to wear; hide hips	need shoulder pads to balance shoulders to hips	need shoulder pads to balance shoulders to hips	need shoulder pads to balance shoulders to hips
▽	be less flattering	balance hips to shoulders; only works if waist is small	make hips look as wide as shoulders	hide full bust and torso; spotlight trim hips
⋈	hide best feature— small waist	emphasize curved shape & smaller waistline	hide best feature— small waist	minimize hips by adding shoulder padding
▭	create an illusion of hip curves	emphasize thick waist	hide thick waist	create a pleasing shape by accenting shoulders

You can use outside lines to make parts of your body look smaller by making other parts look larger. Consider this optical illusion:

Lines X and Y are equal.
Lines A and B are equal.

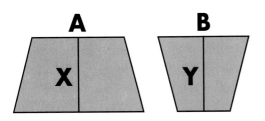

When the lines taper inward from shoulder to waist, the whole body appears more tall and slender. But when the lines from shoulder to waist taper outward the figure looks shorter and the waist fuller.

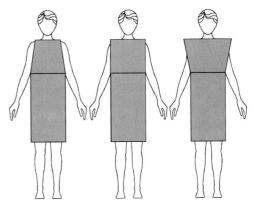

But notice that when the outside lines taper outward, the figure looks shorter. When the outside lines taper in, the figure looks taller. And line B looks smaller than line A.

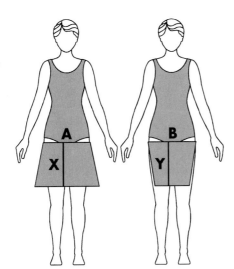

The shoulder line is one of the most critical points of design. Every body type is enhanced by a strong shoulder line.

Now position those shapes over a skirt area. Which shape makes the figure appear taller and the hipline appear narrower? What a convincing argument for tapered skirts and pants!

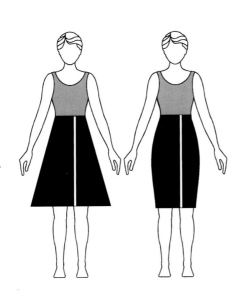

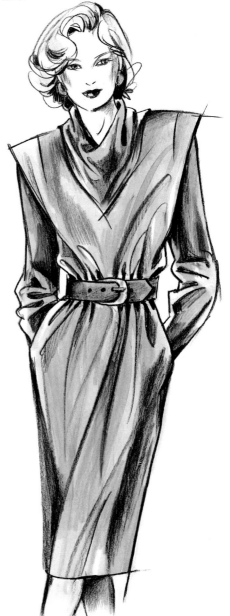

The same illusion illustrates the importance of creating a strong shoulder line with design details or shoulder pads.

Inside Lines

Inside lines move the eye up and down or across your body. They include items like:

♦ Lapels and collars

♦ Detail seams like yokes, princess seams

♦ Pleats, gathers and tucks

♦ Plackets

♦ Rows of buttons

♦ Placement of trims or embroidery

♦ Patch or angled pockets

♦ Topstitching

♦ Color contrasts

♦ Belts or sashes

♦ Details like epaulets, pocket flaps

They can be bold or subtle. The harder you have to look to see them, the less they will affect your appearance.

Notice the inside lines of these garments. They fall into four categories:

Vertical lines lengthen and narrow.

Horizontal lines shorten and widen.

Curved lines add roundness. Vertical curves can lengthen; horizontal curves widen.

Diagonals camouflage by moving the eye indirectly. Near-vertical diagonals lengthen; near-horizontal diagonals widen.

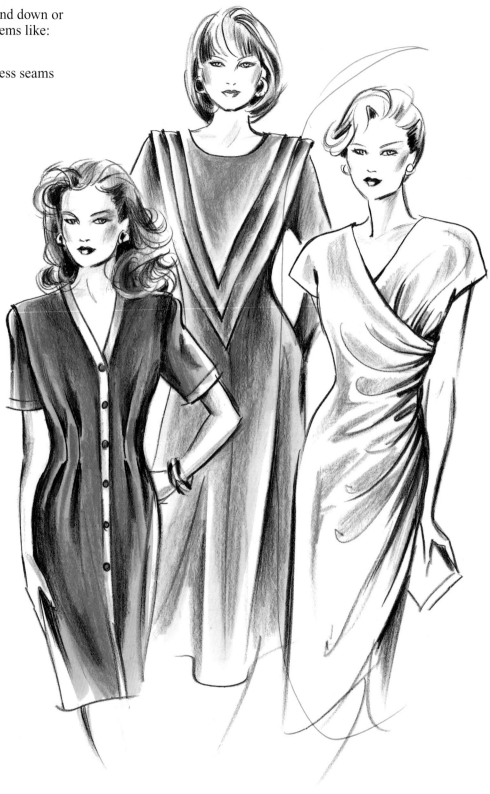

Let's look at some inside lines in action:

Verticals

An unbroken area looks larger than the same area divided into segments by a vertical line. Which figure appears slimmer and taller?

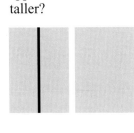

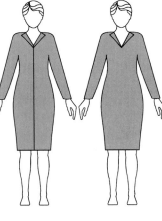

However, not all verticals are created equal. For example:

Which of these equal rectangles appears wider?

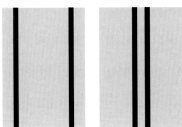

Two verticals placed near the center of the figure draw the eye lengthwise to lengthen and slenderize.

But when the verticals are farther apart, the eye jumps back and forth between them in a (widening) horizontal direction.

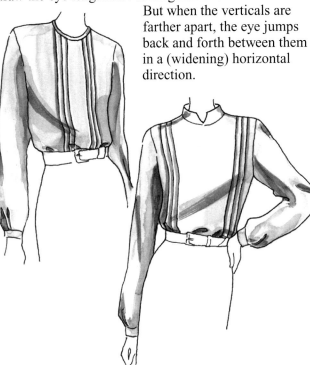

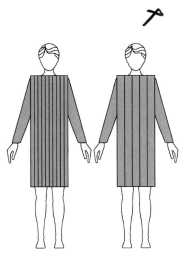

Which of these rectangles appears wider?

A series of many vertical lines (like stripes or pleats) is more slenderizing if they are spaced more closely together.

Which of these equal lines appears longer?

A vertical line lengthens even more when the surrounding lines elongate it. A V neck combined with a center vertical is very slimming.

In contrast, an empire seam or raglan sleeve detail can reduce the lengthening power of the center vertical.

Which of these skirts is more flattering?

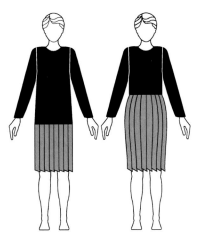

Verticals are more slimming when they fall straight rather than bowing out over body curves. Bowing adds visual width, so most pleats should be stitched to the hip or fall from a yoke.

Horizontals

An unbroken area looks narrower than an equal area divided by a horizontal line.

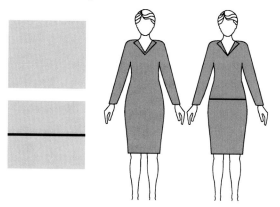

Two horizontals used together widen even more than a single one.

But a series of narrow, evenly spaced horizontals can actually draw the line in an upward direction (climbing the ladder) and create a lengthening effect.

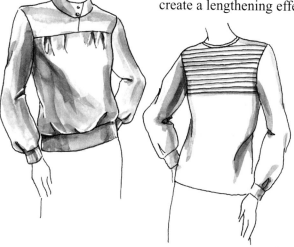

But not all horizontals are equal either.

Because a horizontal tends to hold attention, use one at a place you want to accent or enlarge.

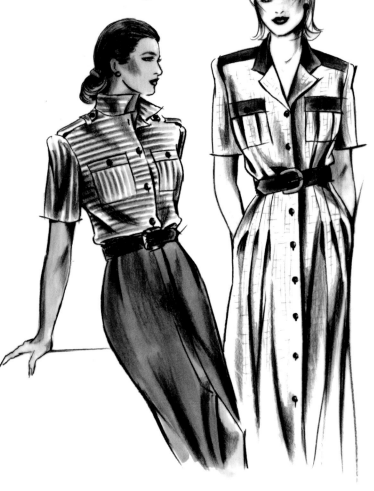

Horizontals placed high or low on the body can slenderize the overall look compared with a horizontal that divides the figure evenly. The longer the eye moves up or down before meeting the horizontal, the taller and slimmer the figure will look.

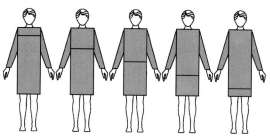

With these ideas about horizontal and vertical lines, which is more figure flattering—tailored trousers or jeans?

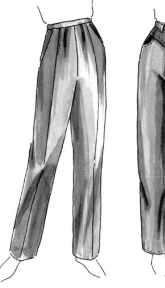

Diagonals

Diagonal lines can be very flattering because they divert the direction of the eye past bust, waist or hips without stopping. The nearer a diagonal is to a vertical direction, the greater its slenderizing power.

At the right are some examples of garments with figure-flattering diagonals.

Plaid fabrics are made up of vertical and horizontal lines. But cut on the bias, they become diagonals and are often much more figure-friendly.

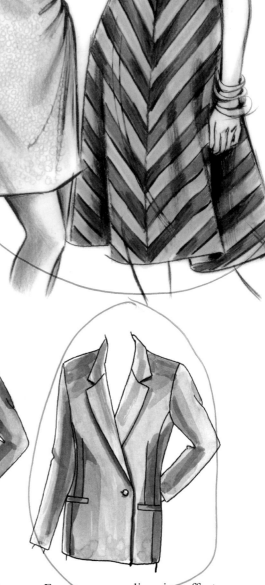

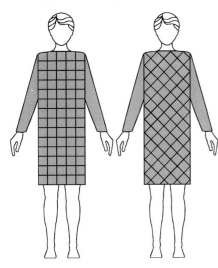

Understanding verticals, horizontals and diagonals, you can improve the slimming potential of a double-breasted jacket.

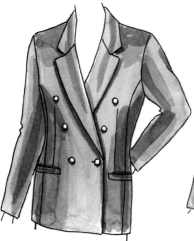

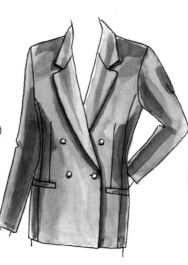

The widely spaced buttons draw the eye from side to side and widen the body.

Remove the nonfunctional top set of buttons.

For even more slimming effect, remove all but one button, creating an asymmetrical closure.

Curves

Curves are gentle, feminine lines, enhancing to most figures. They can add roundness to the figure and create the illusion of more weight on a too-thin frame. The eye will follow a line until it ends or changes direction. Therefore, a line curving upward will make the figure appear taller, while a line curving downward will visually shorten.

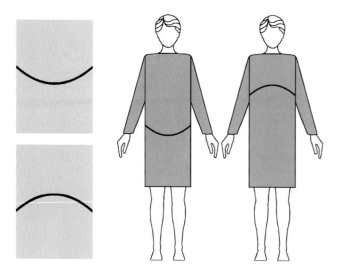

Converging/Diverging

Inside lines can also affect appearance when they come together (converge) or move apart (diverge). The area where the lines meet appears smaller; where they separate appears larger.

Hemlines

Hemlines are horizontals that tend to stop the eye. Be sure they fall at flattering points on your body.

Fortunately, fashion has moved away from rigidly dictated lengths. When it comes to hemlines, we are actively "pro choice." But remember that the fuller the pant or skirt style, the longer it must be to avoid looking boxy.

To determine the flattering lengths for you—

♦ Stand in front of a full-length mirror in underwear and your usual shoes. Hold a large scarf or piece of fabric in front of you, draped to the floor.

♦ Raise and lower the fabric. As the "hem" moves, notice how your legs look.

♦ Identify a flattering length slightly below the knee for shorter, tapered skirts.

♦ Find a second flattering length below the full part of the calf for longer or fuller styles.

♦ Identify any other flattering lengths you see.

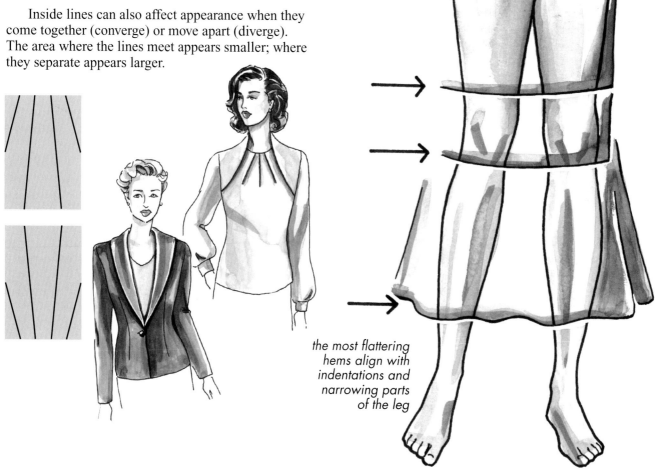

the most flattering hems align with indentations and narrowing parts of the leg

Though hem preferences vary, often one length will be more flattering than another.

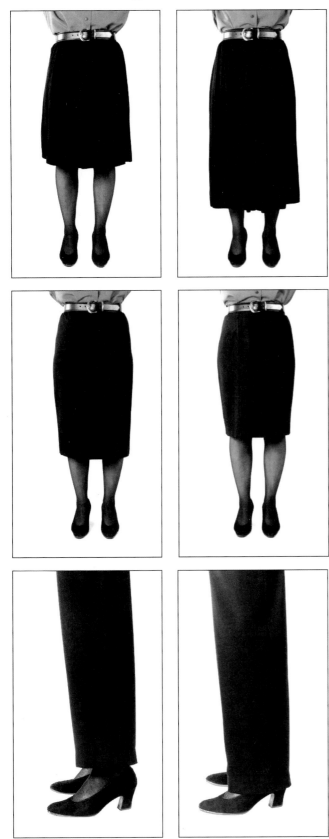

Repeat this exercise with other shoes until you have tried all the heel heights you regularly wear.

Jacket Hems

Avoid a jacket hemmed to the fullest part of your hip unless you need to look wider in **that area.**

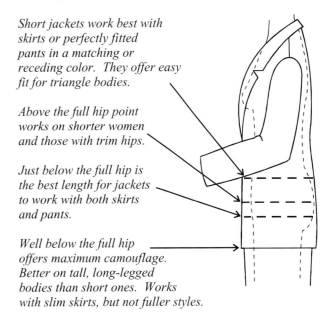

Short jackets work best with skirts or perfectly fitted pants in a matching or receding color. They offer easy fit for triangle bodies.

Above the full hip point works on shorter women and those with trim hips.

Just below the full hip is the best length for jackets to work with both skirts and pants.

Well below the full hip offers maximum camouflage. Better on tall, long-legged bodies than short ones. Works with slim skirts, but not fuller styles.

Pant Hems

The longer the pant leg, the longer your legs will look. Heel height drastically affects pant length and total look, so try on pants with the shoes you plan to wear. Walk around a bit before marking the hem because some pants pull up slightly when worn.

Narrower legs have to be shorter; they can't fit down over the foot.

Straight legs can touch the shoe in front and angle down slightly in back.

Fuller legs can be hemmed nearly to the floor.

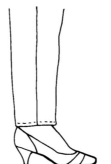
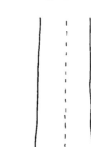
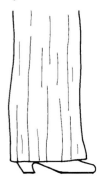

Cuffed pants must be as long as possible, because the cuff forms a visually shortening horizontal. Petites should avoid cuffed pants altogether.

Remember to elongate the look of any pants hemline by matching the color tone of the shoes and hose or socks to the color tone of the garment.

Color

Color can dramatically affect visual body proportions. Notice how the white circle looks larger than the black one in the diagram below.

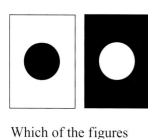

Which of the figures at the right looks more bottom-heavy?

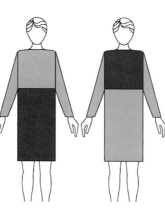

Darker, more subdued colors make the areas they cover appear smaller. Use them to camouflage or minimize body areas. Lighter, brighter colors tend to advance and enlarge. Use them to emphasize assets or increase smaller body areas.

Also notice how your attention goes to the points on the diagram where the color changes from black to white. That "color break" is an attention-getter.

Take care to position color breaks at body areas you want to emphasize.

This light overblouse ending right at the hipline adds unwanted visual pounds. Tucked in and belted it emphasizes a trim waistline instead.

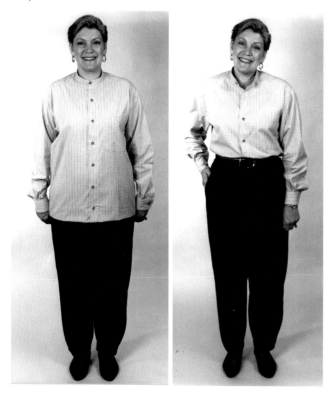

Color contrast can also increase or decrease the impact of inside lines. Notice how the abrupt color change maximizes the impact of the horizontal, while the more subtle color change minimizes it. In an all-one-color suit the jacket's horizontal hemline would virtually disappear.

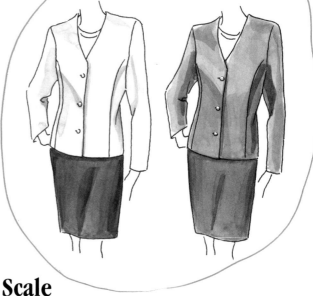

Scale

The balance among various elements affects visual size. Which of the center circles looks larger? Both are the same size, but the one surrounded by smaller dots looks larger than the one surrounded by bigger dots.

Using that concept carefully, you can minimize body size by adding slightly upscaled accessories or using slightly larger print fabrics.

But carried too far, this concept creates visual imbalance. Rectangles A and C look larger due to to the tiny dot pattern. The dots in D are so bold they look out of proportion with the rectangle. B's slightly enlarged dots are the most slenderizing.

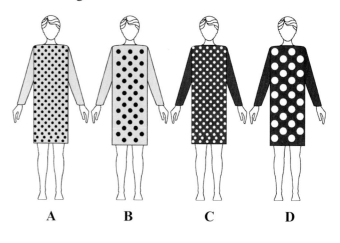

A   B   C   D

Proportion

The relative proportion of color or design elements can make or break a look. A balanced 50:50 ratio is usually dull and uninspiring.

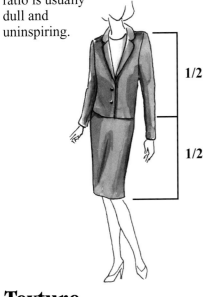

1/2

1/2

Unbalanced proportions are more pleasing to the eye. For example, try pairing a short jacket with a longer skirt or trousers. A longer jacket works best over a very short or very long skirt, not a mid-length one.

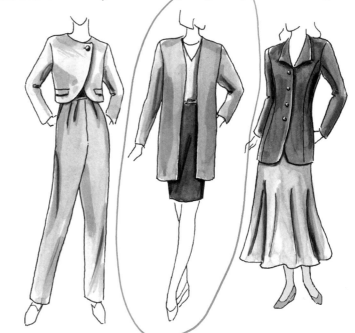

Texture

The look and feel of various fabrics can create proportional illusions too. Very textured, crisp or shiny fabrics can increase visual bulk. Smooth, soft, matte fabrics minimize.

Texture	Effect	Fabric Examples
Very soft and clingy	Follow body curves closely; too revealing for many figures	Single knits, silk jersey, chiffon, crepe de chine, charmeuse
Soft and drapable	Fall softly over curves; slimming in soft styles	Challis, georgette, lightweight gabardine, tissue faille, wool jersey, Ultrasuede Light™ interlock knit
Moderately crisp	Hold garment shape away from body; flatter most because they don't cling	Dress linen, double knit, brushed denim, chino, gabardine, flannel, Ultrasuede® brand fabric
Very crisp	Stand away from body and enlarge the figure	Linen suiting, heavier pique, heavy denim, satin, taffeta
Bulky, coarse, fuzzy	Enlarge the figure; can overpower a petite frame	Tweeds, sweater knits, velour, wide-wale corduroy
Smooth	Flattering to most figures	Gabardine, chino, challis, broadcloth
Shiny	Reflects light and increases body size	Satin, charmeuse, metallic
Dull, matte	Absorbs light and minimizes body size	Matte jersey, flannel, gabardine, interlock knit

CHAPTER 2

Make the Most of Your Body

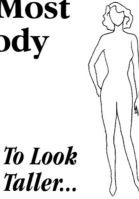

Here are some specific guidelines for applying these concepts to figure challenges women face.

To Look Taller...

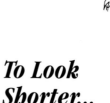

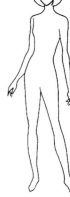

DO

♦ Create a longer line with verticals like front plackets, V necklines, open jackets, trousers.

♦ Wear similar color values from head to toe to create a continuous lengthwise flow.

♦ Color-blend shoes and hose to avoid a distracting color break. When possible, blend both to hemline color.

♦ Choose fuller skirts only in soft, flowing fabrics and longer lengths.

♦ Select shoes with at least 1" heels, even in casual styles.

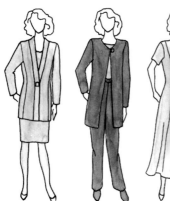

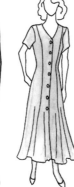

DON'T

♦ Create distracting horizontals with color contrast between jacket, skirt and/or hose.

♦ Use horizontal details like hip yokes, trouser cuffs, bold pocket flaps or border-print hemlines.

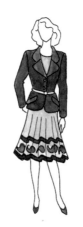

To Look Shorter...

DO

♦ Create horizontal emphasis with hip yokes, pocket flaps, trouser cuffs, wide lapels, bold belts and horizontal stripes.

♦ Select contrasting colors for top and bottom garments.

♦ Keep garment details and accessories medium to bold in scale.

♦ Choose fuller, sweeping styles like capes, swing coats and long, flared skirts.

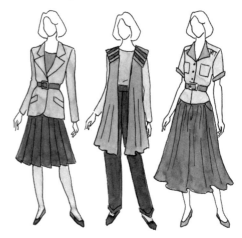

DON'T

♦ Choose styles with too many vertical design lines or one-color outfits head to toe.

♦ Use accessories, details or prints that are too tiny for your body scale.

♦ Ever, ever wear pants or long sleeves that are too short.

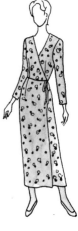

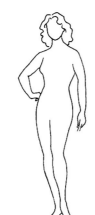

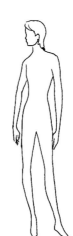

To Look Thinner...

DO

- ♦ Use vertical design lines to lengthen and slenderize.

- ♦ Match or blend colors head to toe, including shoes and hose.

- ♦ Choose medium and dark colors, with bright accents near the face to create a focal point.

- ♦ Strengthen your shoulder line with shoulder pads to balance lower body fullness.

- ♦ Taper slim skirts and pants for a narrower line.

- ♦ Select longer skirts in soft, drapable fabrics.

- ♦ Try fluid, wrap styles that skim over the body and form graceful diagonal lines.

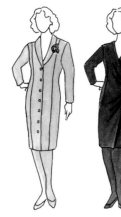 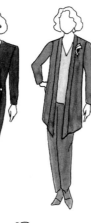

DON'T

- ♦ Use widening horizontal lines lower than shoulder level.

- ♦ Wear anything too baggy (looks sloppy) or too tight (accentuates weight).

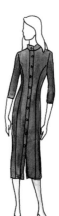

To Look Heavier...

DO

- ♦ Choose horizontal details like yokes, bold belts, stripes, pocket flaps, trouser cuffs.

- ♦ Use gathers and soft fullness to create the illusion of added body bulk.

- ♦ Look for bulky or highly textured fabrics like sweater knits, velour, tweeds, wide-wale corduroy.

- ♦ Use multiple layers to create fashion interest and body fullness.

- ♦ Color-contrast top and bottom garments.

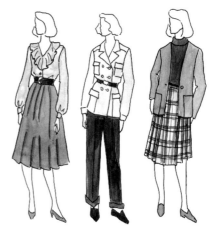

DON'T

- ♦ Use too many vertical design lines.

- ♦ Wear clothes too tight (exposes thinness) or too baggy (you'll look lost).

- ♦ Choose clingy fabrics or body-hugging styles.

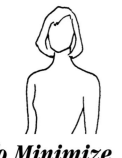
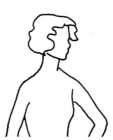
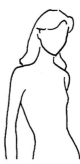

To Minimize Broad/Squared Shoulders...

DO

- Think twice...this is usually a fashion asset!

- Choose raglan styles to create a sloping line.

- Create a center-torso vertical with a V neckline, open jacket, long, narrow lapels or placket detail.

- Create a center-body focal point with a center-tied scarf or a prominent neckline pin.

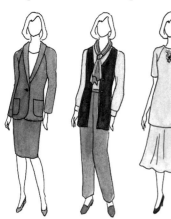

DON'T

- Choose puffed sleeves or wide ruffled collars.

- Add shoulder details like yokes or epaulets.

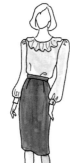

To Broaden Narrow/Sloping Shoulders...

DO

- Make a good pair of shoulder pads your fashion "best friend."

- Select details like yokes, epaulets, bateau necklines, set-in sleeves or wide collars to maintain a horizontal shoulder emphasis.

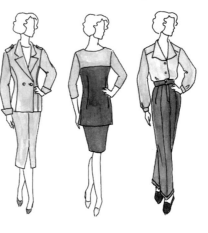

DON'T

- Choose raglan-sleeve styles or halter tops.

- Select tent or swing styles that flare out from the shoulder line.

To Enhance a Small Bust...

DO

- Use layered tops to create visual fullness (sweater over shirt over turtleneck, for example).

- Wear bodices in lighter, brighter colors, with horizontal trims and breast pockets.

- Look for blouses with tucks, ruffles, soft draping or blouson styling.

- Select short vests and bolero-style jackets.

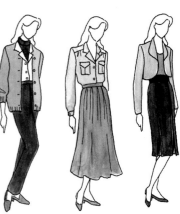

DON'T

- Wear blouse styles that are tight-fitting or too low-cut.

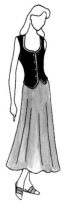

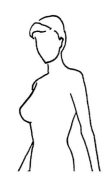
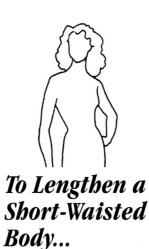
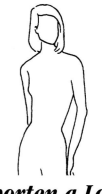

To Minimize a Full Bust...

DO

- Invest in superbly fitted support or minimizer bras.
- Use natural-looking shoulder pads for balance.
- Shift focus upward with interesting necklines, scarves or jewelry. Or lower the focus with colorful skirt prints.
- Choose tapering jackets or over-blouses that end below full hip.
- Try blouson styles with just enough fabric to skim over body fullness.

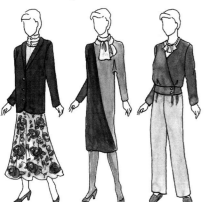

DON'T

- Use horizontal bodice details like breast pockets or short sleeves with contrasting cuffs.
- Choose tight or clingy styles or wide belts or waistbands.

To Lengthen a Short-Waisted Body...

DO

- Conceal the natural waist with dropped, raised or no-waistline styles.
- Choose jackets or blouses that cover or blouse over the waist.
- Try skirt and pant styles with waist facings instead of bands.
- Match belt color to bodice rather than bottoms.

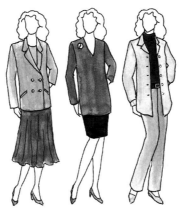

DON'T

- Use horizontal bodice details (yokes, pockets) that visually shorten torso.
- Select full skirts that balloon out from the waist.

To Shorten a Long-Waisted Body...

DO

- Choose shorter jackets in bold, advancing colors, often with horizontal details in the lapels, pockets and trim.
- Use lengthening vertical details on the lower body for balance.
- Try raised-waistline skirt/pant styles, or wider waistbands.
- Color-match belts to trousers or skirt, not to bodice.

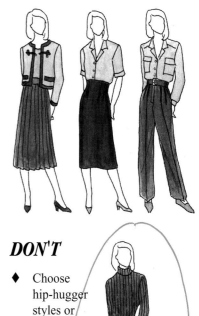

DON'T

- Choose hip-hugger styles or faced waistlines instead of bands.

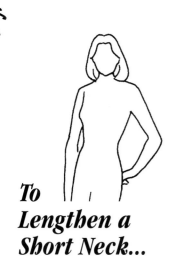

To Lengthen a Short Neck...

DO

♦ Wear V necklines or open collars to elongate the neck.

♦ Keep earrings close to the ear, not dangling.

♦ Wear longer necklaces to expose more neckline area.

♦ Keep hairstyles short or upswept.

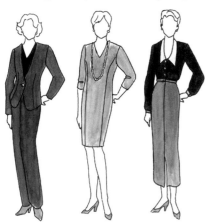

DON'T

♦ Wear turtlenecks or other high necklines.

♦ Choose choker necklaces or tie scarves high on the neck.

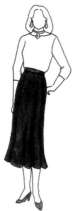

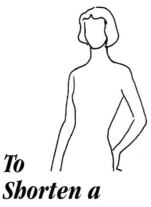

To Shorten a Long Neck...

DO

♦ Realize that a long neck is often a fashion asset.

♦ Enjoy the ability to wear turtlenecks, choker necklaces and other accessories close to the neck.

♦ Fill in the neckline area with longer, fuller hair.

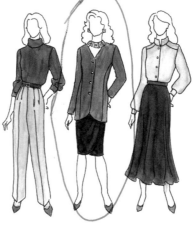

DON'T

♦ Exaggerate the length with severe V necks in garments or jewelry.

♦ Choose earring styles that are very long and narrow.

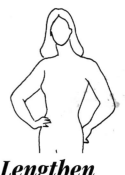

To Lengthen or Slenderize Arms...

DO

♦ Create the longest possible line from shoulder to wrist with tapered set-in sleeves or raglan styles.

♦ Use shoulder pads and details like epaulets to further enhance length.

♦ Keep cuffs moderate in size and color-matched to sleeve.

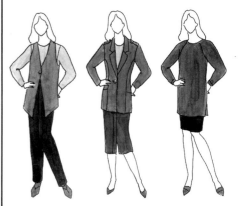

DON'T

♦ Choose sleeves that are either too tight or too full.

♦ Wear short sleeves, especially ones with fitted cuffs.

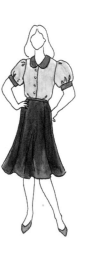

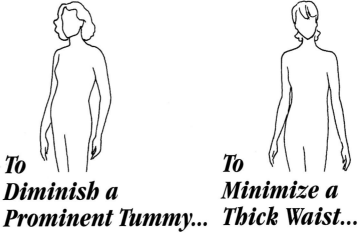

To Camouflage Long, Thin Arms...

DO

- Choose horizontal sleeve details like puffed, drop-shoulder, push-up or short, cuffed sleeves.
- Find long sleeves with wide or contrasting cuffs.
- Be sure long sleeves are not too short; alter if necessary.

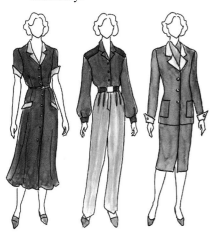

DON'T

- Wear raglan-sleeve styling.
- Choose very tight sleeves.

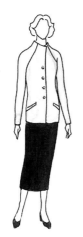

To Diminish a Prominent Tummy...

DO

- Create a prominent shoulder line with shoulder pads, yokes, wide lapels or horizontal collar styles.
- Wear styles that skim over the abdomen and taper at the hemline.
- Wear cardigans, swing jackets or shirt-jackets that conceal the abdomen. Pair them with tapered skirts or pants.
- Try longer blouson tops softly banded or tied below the tummy.
- Choose gently gathered skirts in soft fabrics.

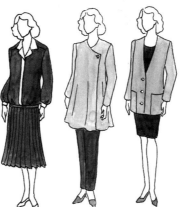

DON'T

- Use bulky, stiff or shiny fabrics on the lower body.
- Choose front closure styles, full gathers, trouser pockets and bold belts.

To Minimize a Thick Waist...

DO

- Keep belts and waistbands narrow and inconspicuous.
- Look for straight, body-skimming styles that obscure the waist, tapered at the hemline.
- Choose semifitted jackets with shoulder emphasis for balance. Wear them unbuttoned, for a slenderizing vertical band of blouse color underneath.
- Try a decorative belt buckle, worn under an unbuttoned jacket for a center-body focal point.

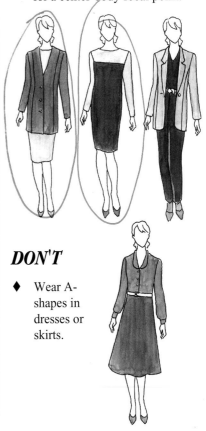

DON'T

- Wear A-shapes in dresses or skirts.

To Lengthen Short Legs...

DO

- Keep skirt lengths flattering; just below the knee and just below the full calf are safe spots.
- Choose trouser styles with vertical details like fly-front closure, pleats, and/or creases.
- Look for skirts and pants with wider waistbands to elongate the look.
- Create an upward focus with bright tops and eye-catching jewelry.

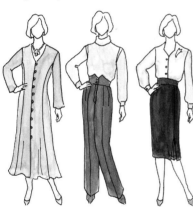

DON'T

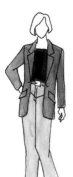

- Wear pants/skirts with horizontal details (cuffs, yokes, patch pockets, border prints).

To Shorten Long Legs...

DO

- Wear sweaters, tunics or blouses that end at high hip or mid-thigh.
- Match belt color to top garment, not skirt or pants.
- Choose pants with horizontal yokes, faced waistlines and cuffs.
- Hem fuller skirts to mid-calf length.

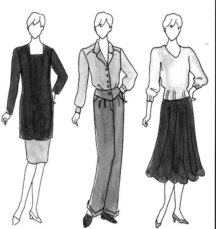

DON'T

- Tuck fitted blouses into high-rise waistlines.

To Enhance Narrow Hips/Derriere...

DO

- Choose flared or gathered skirts in moderately crisp fabrics.
- Try jackets with peplums or swing styles to add hipline fullness.

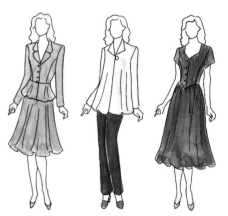

DON'T

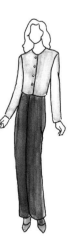

- Wear pants or skirts with baggy fullness below the derriere. Alter if necessary for proper fit.

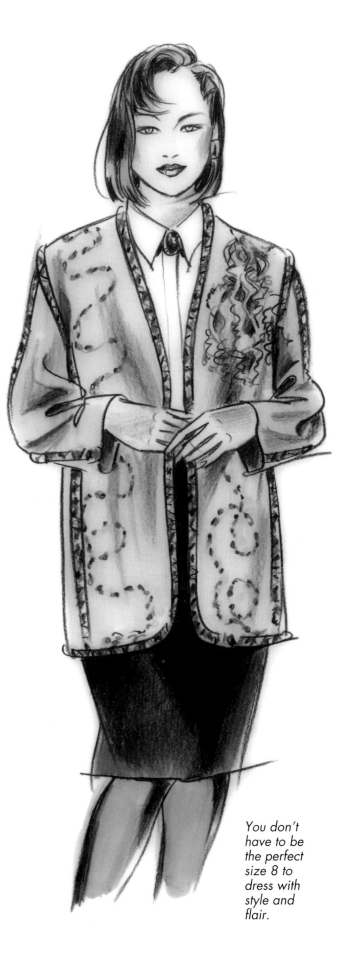

To Slenderize Heavy Hips/ Thighs/Derriere...

DO

♦ Broaden shoulders with shoulder pads and wide collars to balance hips.

♦ Use brightly colored tops with eye-catching details to focus attention on the upper body.

♦ Select dark-colored skirts or pants that skim over the hips and taper at the hemline for a narrower look.

♦ Look for skirts with center-front pleats or plackets to draw the eye toward the center of the figure.

♦ Choose jackets that end above or below the widest part of hips.

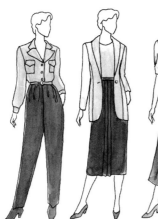

DON'T

♦ Position any eye-catching details at the hipline (yokes, pockets).

♦ Wear pants too tight, creating horizontal wrinkles. Buy to fit the hips and alter the waist.

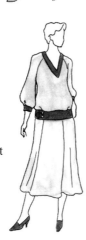

You don't have to be the perfect size 8 to dress with style and flair.

CHAPTER 3

Underneath It All: The Inside Story

Of course outer garments can look only as good as the garments worn under them. Body lumps and bumps can ruin the look of the loveliest dress. And a sagging bustline adds 10 pounds and 10 years to a woman's figure.

Bras

A properly fitted bra can minimize a full bustline or enhance a smaller one. But many women mistakenly buy a too-large bra size with a too-small cup. The result is breast tissue slipping out below the band and overflowing the cup at the neckline and armhole.

Take a snug under-bust measurement and add 5 to determine your correct *bra* size. Then subtract the underbust number from the full-bust measurement to determine *cup* size:

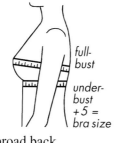

0" difference	. . . A cup
1" difference	. . . B cup
2" difference	. . . C cup
3" difference	. . . D cup
4" difference	. . . DD cup

full-bust

under-bust +5 = bra size

Women who have a broad back may find that this formula doesn't work well for them. Professional help may solve the problem. Few department stores today have professionals trained to help customers fit undergarments accurately. Check your Yellow Pages for lingerie specialty stores. Or see our resource guide on page 155.

To put on a bra, bend from the waist as you slip your arms through the straps so the breasts literally pour into the cups, above the band. Hook the back of the bra below the shoulder blades, then stand upright. Adjust the straps so the bust point falls midway between the sternal notch (the small hollow at the base or your neck) and the navel.

Choose a bra—and other undergarments—in a color near your skin tone to minimize shadowing through lightweight clothes.

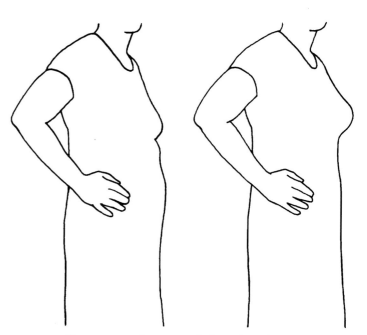

Change your silhouette with the right undergarments.

Panties

Briefs, bikinis or scantier styles can all work well, provided they are large enough not to cut into soft flesh, making unsightly bulges under clothing. A cotton-lined crotch is important for air flow to prevent infections.

Many women substitute panty hose for panties. Other women wear both.

Control-top panty hose provide a measure of tummy control. Choose a brand that diminishes its level of control gradually from waistline to midthigh. An abrupt end to the control element causes uncomfortable binding and an unattractive bump.

When you find a brand of panty hose you love, stock up on all your basic colors, then

desk drawer ?

keep a spare pair in your desk drawer and another in your car's glove compartment for emergencies.

Keep panty hose with minor runs to wear under pants, but tie them in a soft knot after laundering so you can identify them in your lingerie drawer.

On the inevitable day when you have no run-free pairs in the needed color, try this trick:

Cut off the leg with the run from two matching pairs. Put one run-free leg on your left side, the other on your right side. If the hose are control-top, you'll get double tummy control too.

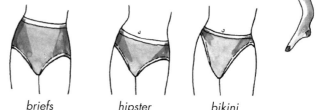

briefs   *hipster*   *bikini*

54

Body Shapers

The reincarnation of the '60s girdle, a body shaper keeps tummy, derriere and thighs looking firmer. Sit down when trying one on because your body will expand 3-6" when seated. If the waistline flips down or the legs creep or curl up, try a larger size.

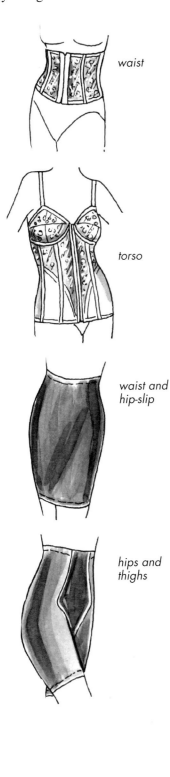

waist

torso

waist and hip-slip

hips and thighs

Swim Shapes

Probably no garment selection process creates more anxiety than shopping for a swimsuit. Any swimsuit reveals a lot about the wearer's body, but certain styles help balance body challenges:

Tummy bulge—look for a suit with an extra tummy-control panel to flatten and a diagonal sarong panel to distract the eye.

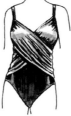

Wide waist— try a color-block suit with a dark color at the waist or in shaped side panels.

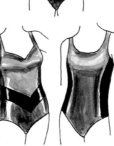

Heavy hips—skip skirted suits; they conceal but add unwanted width. Instead, opt for dark bottoms/light tops with upper body detailing and a moderately high leg cut.

No hips—a ruffled skirt instantly adds the illusion of curves.

Small bust—avoid tank suits that flatten your bosom. Go for gathered or shirred bodices or bust structure like seaming or underwires.

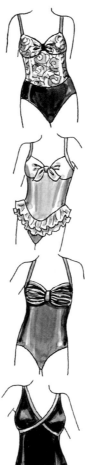

Full bust—insist on a style with under-bust seams or cross-wrap styling and built-in bra cups. Check for adequate cover-age—no spill-over at neckline or armholes.

For overall slimming, look for darker colors, moderately cut legs, bulge-concealing fabric textures or prints, and vertical or diagonal prints or design lines.

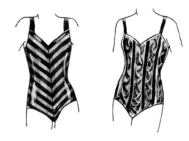

In two-piece styles, a brief that comes to the waistline is more slimming than one that cuts across the full hipline.

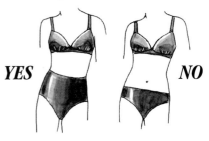

YES   **NO**

Care

Wash undergarments by hand or in a cool-water gentle machine cycle. Use Ivory soap or a special lingerie cleaner. Avoid Woolite, which is made for natural fibers, not synthetics. Heat destroys spandex fibers, so skip the dryer and line dry instead.

Prolong the life of your swimsuit by rinsing it in cool water and mild soap after every wearing. Water alone won't remove salt, chlorine and oils, which destroy spandex fibers. Deteriorated spandex results in broken white threads popping out from the fabric's surface and in stretched-out elastic. Never machine wash or dry a swimsuit, or hang it in the sun to dry.

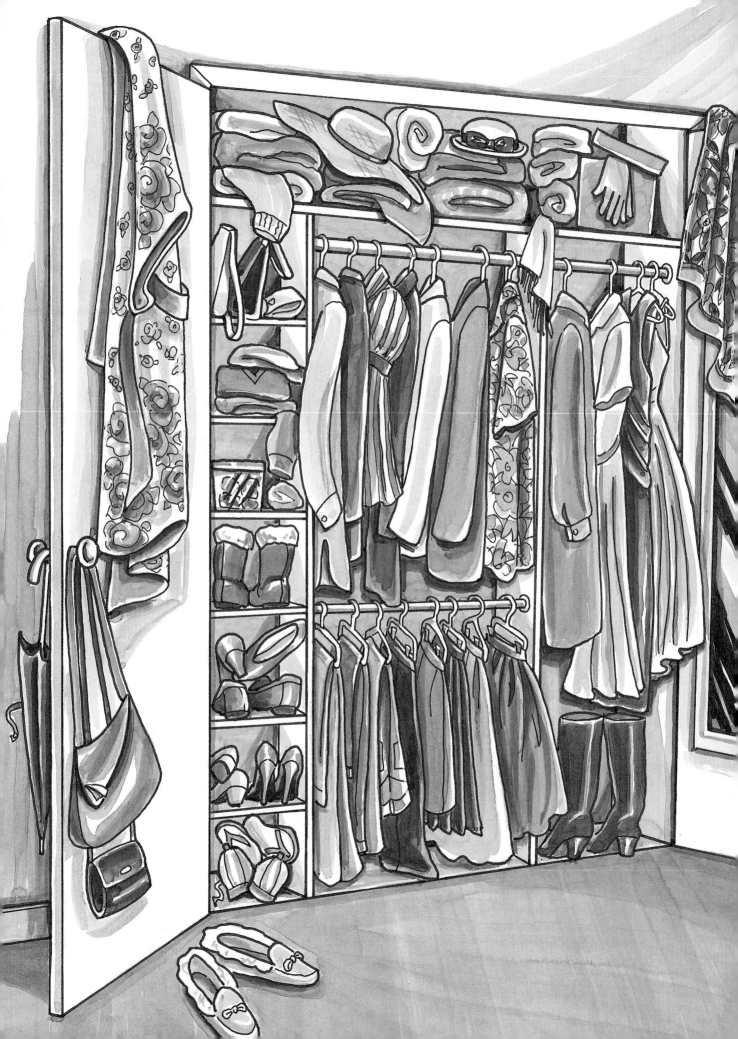

CHAPTER 4

The Wardrobe Workout

Closet Clean-Out

"I never have anything to wear."

If that sounds familiar, there is hope. You **can** learn to spend half the money, own half the clothes...and have twice as much to wear.

Begin by organizing the clothes you already own. Now that you know what colors and styles are most flattering you can easily determine which items should stay and which should go.

Of course it's hard to discard perfectly good clothes. But when you get rid of a garment that doesn't look or feel good, you're making room for one that will.

Make a closet clean-out a seasonal habit. Do one early each season, while the stores have the best selection of things to fill the fashion gaps.

Style your hair and put on makeup. Put on good underwear and pantyhose. You'll be trying everything on...and nothing will look good if YOU look awful.

Ready - Set - Toss

1. Pull everything out of your closet and drawers, the attic, under the bed and wherever else you hide clothes...especially the ones you don't wear.

2. Store away items that won't work for the coming season. Trying to consider an entire year's wardrobe is too overwhelming. Focus just on fall/winter or spring/summer.

3. Try on everything. Admittedly, this is about as much fun as trying on swimsuits in January. But the payoff may be finding unexpected treasures.

4. Evaluate each garment using this point system:

Design lines flattering to my body	2 pts	_____
Fits well OR Can be readily altered to fit	2 pts or 1 pt	_____
Color is enhancing	2 pts	_____
Garment is in good condition	2 pts	_____
Style is still fashionable OR Can be easily updated	2 pts or 1 pt	_____
	TOTAL	_____

Is this item a Yes, No or Maybe?

8-10 points

This is an obvious "YES"—a key part of your new wardrobe plan. If it needs minor repairs, put it in a separate pile labeled "Fix Now." Otherwise, it goes back in the closet.

0-4 points

An equally obvious "NO." This item has to GO. You probably don't wear it anyway. It just takes up valuable closet space and makes you feel guilty about making a shopping mistake. Who needs all that negative energy? Get rid of it fast...before you change your mind.

- Swap with friends. Your trash could be their treasure and vice versa.

- Resale shops will generally pay you 50 percent of the resale price. Clothes must be like new and cleaned/pressed.

- Charitable organizations are the best recipients for worn or out-of-style items. Be sure to get a receipt; your donation is tax deductible.

5-7 points

This is a "Maybe"—the most challenging category. It may be a good candidate for an update. Could you increase its point total to the "Yes" category by:

- Lengthening, shortening or tapering?

- Dyeing it a more flattering color?

- Adding a trim...or removing one?

- Replacing unattractive buttons?

- Combining it with a more flattering garment?

If you can't update, you have a decision to make. Can you afford to toss it, or should you keep it for now and plan to replace it as soon as possible?

Sometimes women keep items because "It might come back in style." Fashions do run in cycles, but they seldom come back quite the same. Our tastes—and our figures—usually change in the interim.

The following items:

Rarely Come Back for Long	Will Always Come Back
shoe styles	most wool sweaters
handbag styles	knee-length skirts
trendy prints	any classic style in a
oversized collars,	very good fabric
lapels, cuffs	(silk, wool, cashmere)

Just can't part with some of your "maybe" items? Put them in a box in the attic and check them again next year. You'll either find an unexpected treasure or a great laugh.

You may also decide you will be a "collector." A collection of historic fashion pieces could one day be valuable...or at least a great nostalgia trip.

Fashion Make-Overs

Don't hesitate to remodel even an expensive garment. Better to refit or restyle an item than to have it hang unworn in the closet gathering dust.

Consider these factors:

1. How much time will the update take (or how much will it cost)?

2. Is the quality of the fabric worth the update investment?

3. Would replacing the item be easier or cheaper?

4. Are seam allowances deep enough to let out? Will pockets or other details get in the way of the alterations?

5. Will original stitching or hemlines show?

We'll concentrate on updating items you already own, but the same techniques can apply to new clothes as well. Sometimes a real bargain just needs minor changes to fit or look like a million.

Chapter 11, "And So You Sew," will give you the sewing techniques you need to accomplish simple make-overs, plus additional make-over ideas. See pages 141-148.

The Simplest Make-Over— Wear It a New Way

♦ Wear a big shirt as a light jacket or a beach coverup.

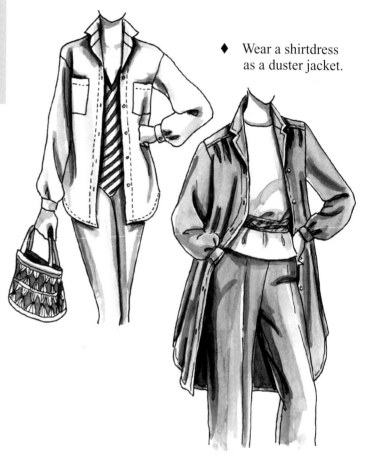

♦ Wear a shirtdress as a duster jacket.

♦ Criss-cross the points of a too-wide collar and anchor with a pretty pin.

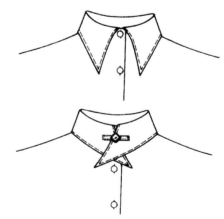

♦ Wear a worn shirt under a crew neck. Tuck in over-sized collar points.

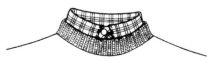

If you need a pro to execute your restyling:

♦ Shop around to find someone you trust. Ask friends for recommendations.

♦ Ask to see samples of the tailor's work. A good one won't be offended.

♦ Ask if fees are hourly or per project. Per project lets you know exactly what you'll spend.

♦ Bring examples from magazines or your closet to show how you want the garment restyled.

♦ Tipping isn't expected, but do compliment a job well done.

Mix, Match and Multiply

When every remaining item in your closet is a "Yes," you're ready to begin coordinating.

Get the Clothes Ready

Group your garments on the closet rods this way:

♦ All one-piece dresses together

♦ All bottoms together (skirts, pants)

♦ All tops together (blouses, jackets, sweaters, vests)

♦ Yes, that means splitting up suits and two-piece dresses so you can see the mix-match potential of each individual piece.

♦ Arrange each grouping in rainbow order:
black—gray—white—beige—brown—red—orange—yellow—green—blue—purple

♦ Pull out all your belts, purses, shoes, scarves and jewelry, even fashion hosiery.

Get You Ready

Style your hair, put on makeup and good underwear. You're going to be in a fashion show.

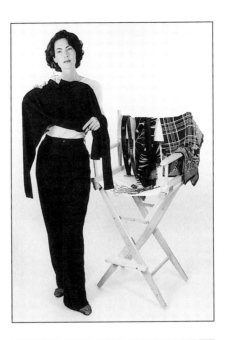

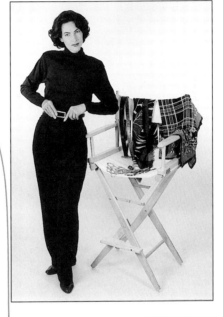

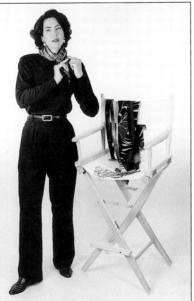

Get Going

Put on the first bottom—perhaps a black wool trouser—then follow this sequence:

Pull out the first top—let's say its a black cotton turtleneck. Hold it up to your body over the black trouser and check the mirror.

Could they be worn together?

If the answer is "No," put it back in the closet and try top #2.

If the answer is "Yes," put on the top. Then work with your accessories to complete the look.

♦ *What shoes and hose would go with it?*

♦ *Does it need a belt?*

♦ *Try scarves and jewelry as accents.*

Use the point system from page 102 to determine if your new outfit is unfinished or overdone. When the whole look works well, list the pieces on a copy of the work sheet (page 63).

If the look needs a finishing touch you don't have, list in the "Need" column.

Now can you create another look by using different accessories with these garments?

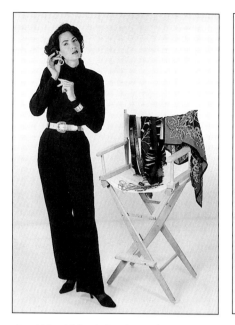

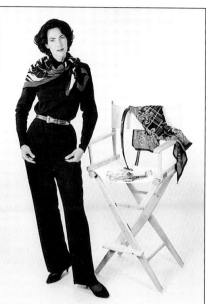

Complete these variations and list them on the work sheet.

♦ *Would high heels and more elegant jewelry give the turtleneck and trousers a dressier look?*

♦ *Could you wear the turtleneck out and belt it?*

Still working with the first top and bottom, look at the other tops in your closet. Are there other pieces you might layer into this combination?

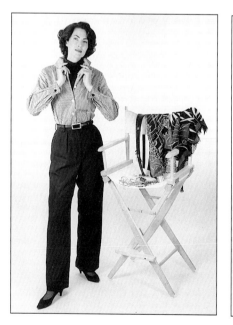

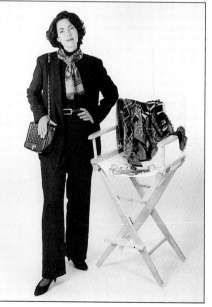

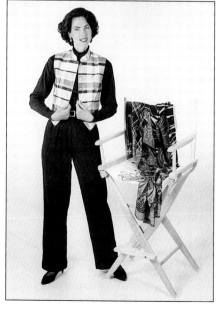

♦ *A shirt to wear over the turtleneck*

♦ *The jacket that matches the trousers*

♦ *A plaid vest*

Wardrobe Work Sheet

BOTTOMS	TOPS — Shirt/Blouse	Jacket/Sweater/Vest	Jewelry/Scarf	ACCESSORIES — Belt/Handbag/Hose/Shoes	NEED
				black belt w/ gold trim buckle black loafer	bold black/gold earring
				"	
black wool trouser	black cotton turtleneck		matte gold earring red/black gold silk scarf	silver belt black suede pump	
"	"		silver loop earring silver bracelet	brown "snakeskin" belt black suede pump	earring?
"	"	over trouser	oversize rayon/cotton scarf – black/brown/cream	black belt w/ gold trim buckle black suede pump	
"	red striped blouse worn over turtleneck	tucked in	black/gold earring oblong paisley silk scarf	" plus black Doncaster bag black belt w/ gold trim buckle black suede pump	
"	black suit jacket		gold drop earring	black belt w/ gold trim buckle black suede pump	low heel black pump
"	plaid silk vest		carnelian earring	"	"
"	red/black stripe knit cardigan			"	
"	red cardigan sweater w/ plaid applique		"		
"	white cotton pleat-front shirt				

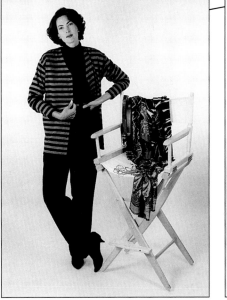

♦ A cardigan knit jacket

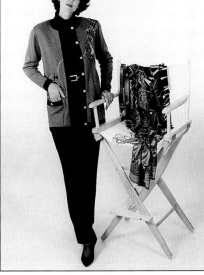

♦ A cardigan sweater

Complete each of these new combinations with accessories and, when they work well, list them on the work sheet.

When you have exhausted the possibilities with bottom #1 and top #1, try that same bottom with top #2 and repeat the cycle. When you've tried every top with that first bottom, try on bottom #2 and start through the tops again.

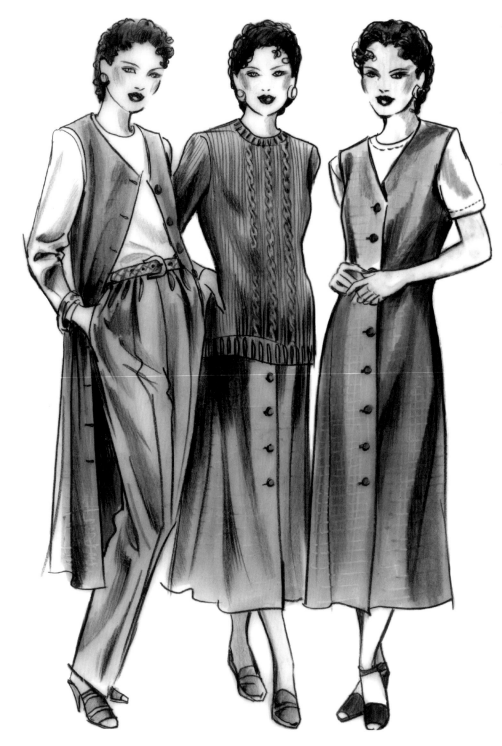

Don't forget the dresses.

♦ *Some can be tops worn as a tunic over pants or layered, unbuttoned, as a long duster jacket.*

♦ *Others can be bottoms, topped with a jacket or sweater.*

♦ *Try layering T-shirts, turtlenecks and blouses under a dress for a new look.*

You'll almost certainly be amazed at the number of combinations you already have. And you'll quickly learn which types of garments are versatile and which are not.

You'll also see certain items appear again and again in the Need column. List those items on your immediate "Needs" shopping list to ensure that you spend your money on the things that will give you the most immediate return.

You may spot Needs in another way as well. If you found a dozen ways to wear that black trouser and only three ways to wear its matching jacket, you could wear out the trouser too fast.

You might invest in a black skirt. Or you could buy another bottom to wear with the jacket—a black-and-red challis pleated skirt could be a good choice in our example, especially if you had several red tops.

Wardrobe Work Sheet

| BOTTOMS | TOPS | | ACCESSORIES | | NEED |
	Shirt/Blouse	Jacket/Sweater/Vest	Jewelry/Scarf	Belt/Handbag/Hose/Shoes	

Make copies of this page.

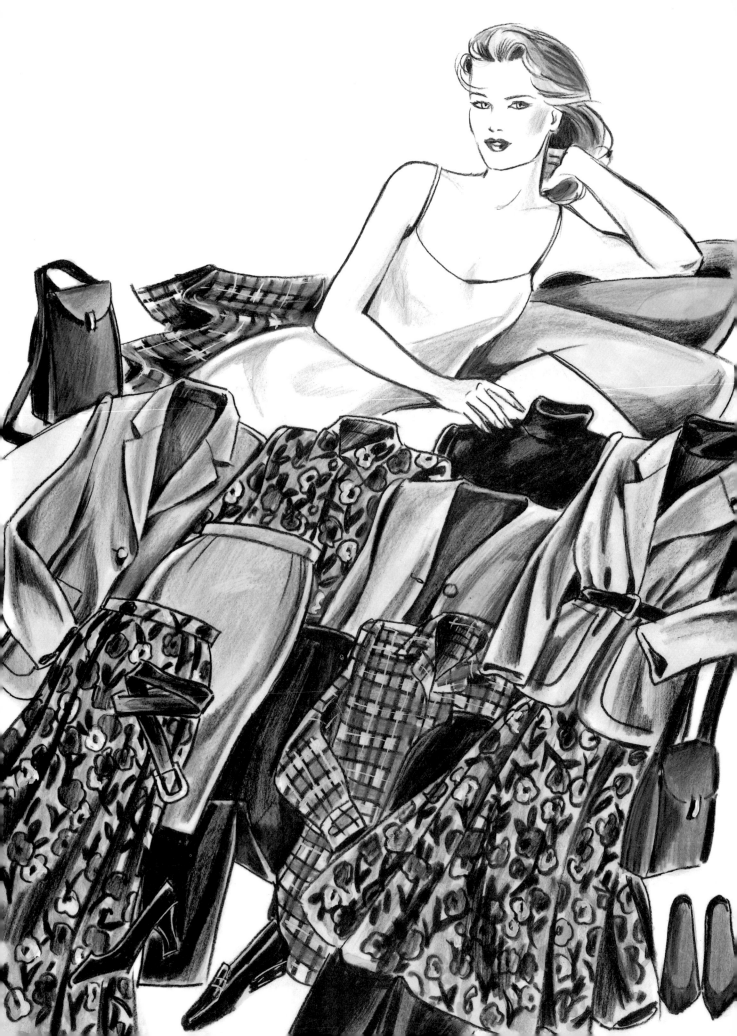

CHAPTER 5

Building Closet Capsules

The Capsule Concept

Building a workable wardrobe is easiest when you think in terms of "closet capsules." No, that's not a pill you take to forget your wardrobe woes!

It simply means building groups of 5-12 related pieces that can be worn in a number of combinations.

There is no single formula for a capsule, but here are some guidelines.

♦ Solid-color pieces mix more readily than patterned ones.

♦ A few print pieces can be the links between diverse solids.

♦ Simple, untrimmed styles are the most versatile, and their classic lines won't look out-of-fashion next year.

♦ Year-round or season-spanning fabric will give you the most use. (This is admittedly easier to accomplish in some climates than others.)

♦ No two items in a capsule should be the same style. You won't get bored with a capsule that contains both trousers and knit pants, both a short, slim skirt and a longer, pleated style, etc.

♦ Forget the idea that everything has to go with everything. That's just too restrictive. Instead, insist that each piece work with three others.

♦ Every item should be in your most flattering colors and styles. Versatility is worthless if all those combinations don't flatter YOU.

♦ Matching multiple pieces in the same solid color—even black—is very difficult. If a skirt, pants and/or jacket need to match exactly, buy them at the same time from the same manufacturer.

There Are Also a Few Don'ts

♦ Don't select stand-alone items for a capsule. A dress with multicolor braid or a jacket with contrasting piping and buttons won't mix and match well with other pieces.

♦ Don't invest your money in a style that is so "IN" this year that by next year it will look like "last year."

Year 'Round Fabrics:

♦ lightweight wool gabardine and flannel
♦ wool crepe and georgette
♦ wool or rayon challis
♦ rayon-blend gabardine and crepe
♦ wool or silk jersey
♦ silk or linen suitings
♦ silk and silk-like blouse weights
♦ cotton and cotton blend knits
♦ Ultrasuede® and other synthetic suedes
♦ fine-wale corduroy
♦ denim and chino

Year 'Round Colors:

COOL	WARM
black	beige
navy	olive
red	cream
cream	purple
purple	camel
medium gray	cocoa
royal blue	khaki
taupe	red

Start With Your Closet

How do you start to build a capsule? The ideal starting point is the items already in your closet. Let's suppose your closet clean-out turned up a pair of black trousers and a red suit.

◆ You could wear the red jacket with the pants.

◆ Other solids that would work with the red could also go with the black.

◆ YES! These pieces could easily be the start of a capsule.

Step 1

Find a print garment or scarf to tie the two solids together, and perhaps add a third solid. This red-royal-black print works well.

And the two-piece dress is a wonderful wardrobe extender. It looks like a dress when you wear the pieces together, but the top and bottom can split up to work in other ways too. Already we have six combinations.

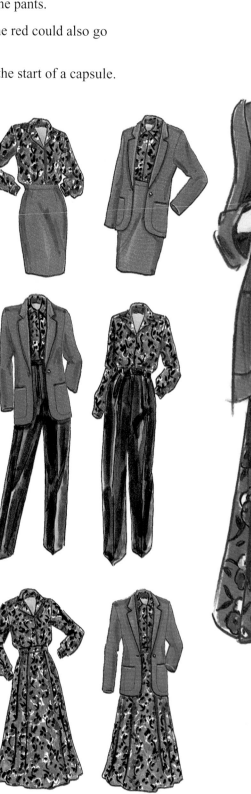

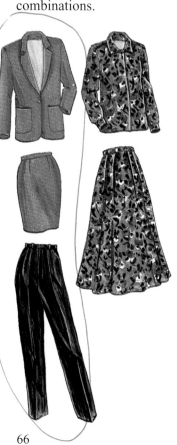

Starting Pieces

66

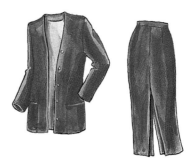

Step 2

Pick another solid color from the print and repeat it in basic pieces. A royal blue skirt and soft knit jacket add eight new looks to this capsule.

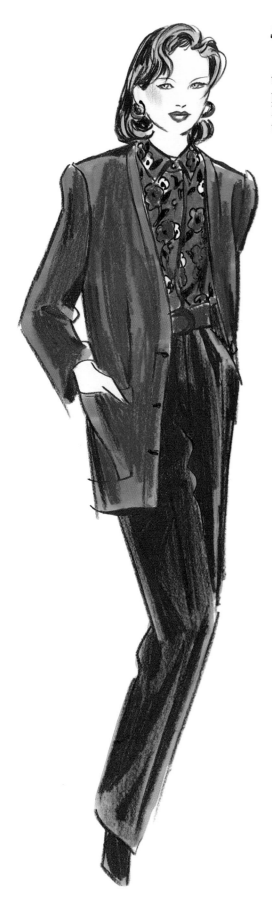

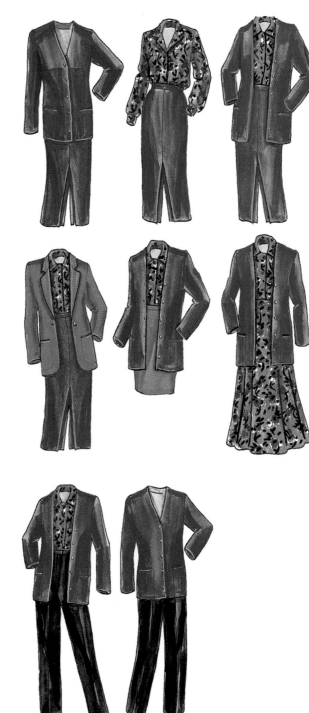

Step 3

Consider other basic pieces that could extend this capsule. Remember the Rule of Three. Each added piece should work at least three ways.

♦ A black turtleneck could work into at least 16 combinations. Can you find them all?

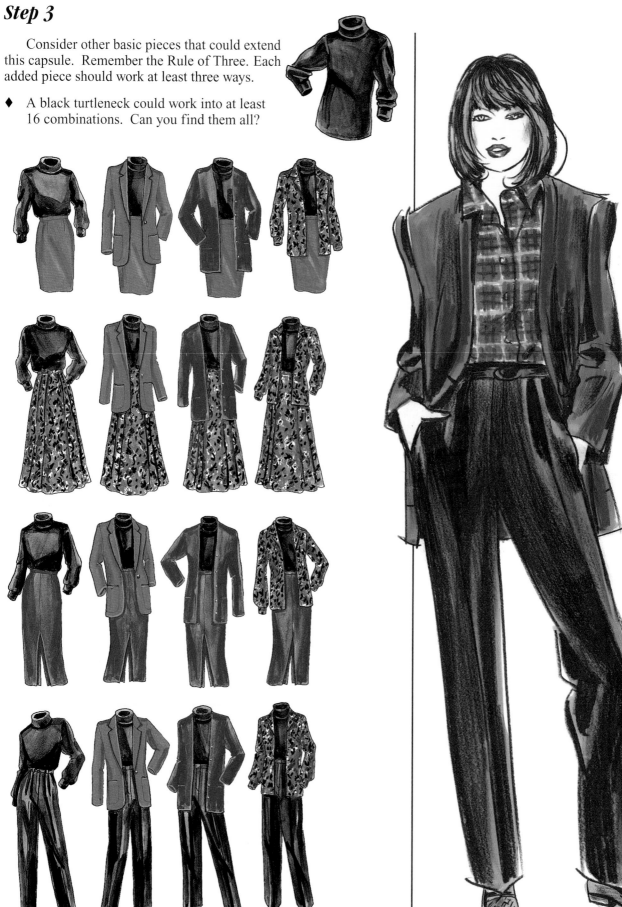

♦ A mini-tartan plaid shirt could be a blouse with any of the solid jackets and bottoms...or function as a jacket when worn over the turtleneck.

That's 12 more combinations. Just think—six well-chosen pieces plus three from the closet add up to 41 different outfits!

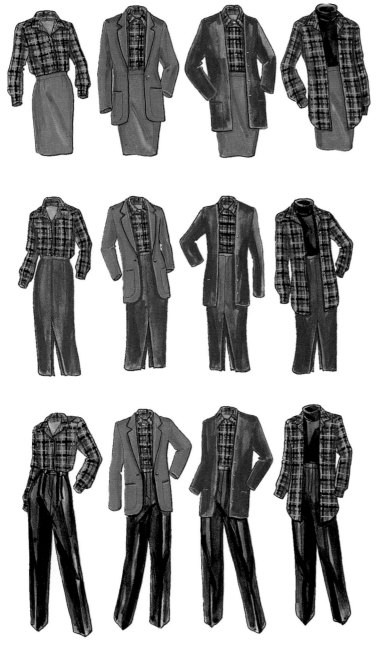

If you are bold, try a print/plaid combination! For more information on combining prints and plaids, see page 82 & 83.

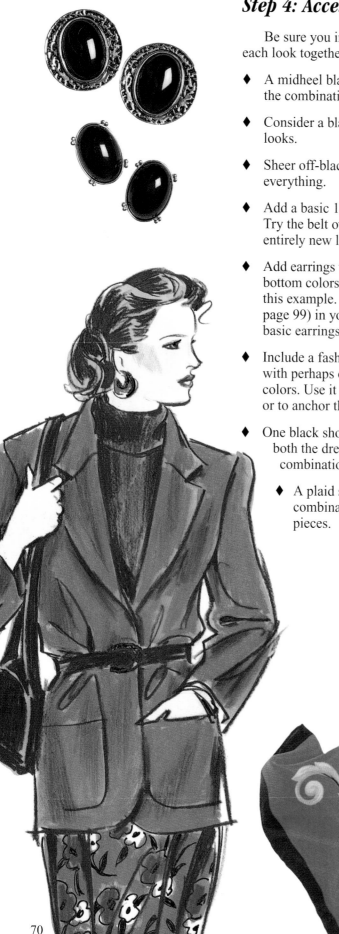

Step 4: Accessories

Be sure you include accessories to pull each look together. You won't need many.

- A midheel black pump works with all the combinations if necessary.

- Consider a black loafer for sportier looks.

- Sheer off-black hose work with everything.

- Add a basic 1" black leather belt. Try the belt over a jacket for an entirely new look.

- Add earrings to coordinate with all the bottom colors—red, royal and black in this example. Earring jackets (see page 99) in your best metal dress the basic earrings up or down.

- Include a fashion pin in your metal— with perhaps one of the wardrobe colors. Use it to dress up the jackets, or to anchor the scarf.

- One black shoulder bag goes with both the dressier and more casual combinations.

- A plaid scarf helps unify combinations of the solid pieces.

Tailor *Your* Capsule to Your Seasonal Colors

Of course you can recolor this sample capsule for your seasonal category:

- Summer—try taupe, cadet blue and mauve

- Spring—consider tan, seafoam green and melon

- Fall—experiment with brown, rust and teal

Photocopy the next page and try out the color combinations that work best for you.

The Basic 9-Piece Capsule in YOUR Colors

Use colored pencils or markers to try out new color combinations.

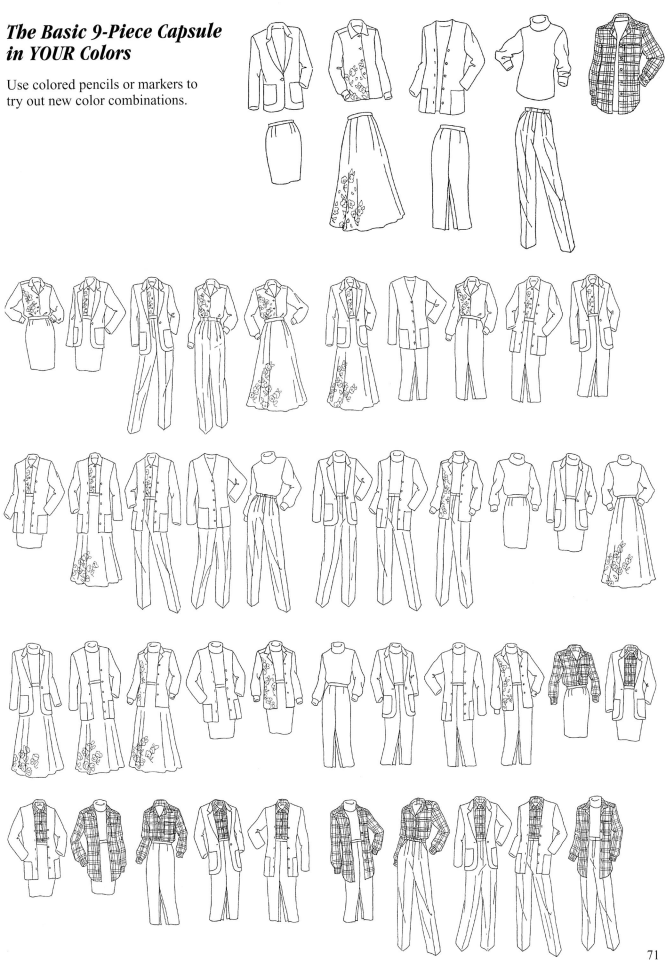

A Second Capsule

WHAT NEXT? Well instead of expanding this capsule further—which could eventually get pretty boring—start another one.

Perhaps you have a couple of basic navy pieces that could be the start of a navy/jade green/fuchsia capsule.

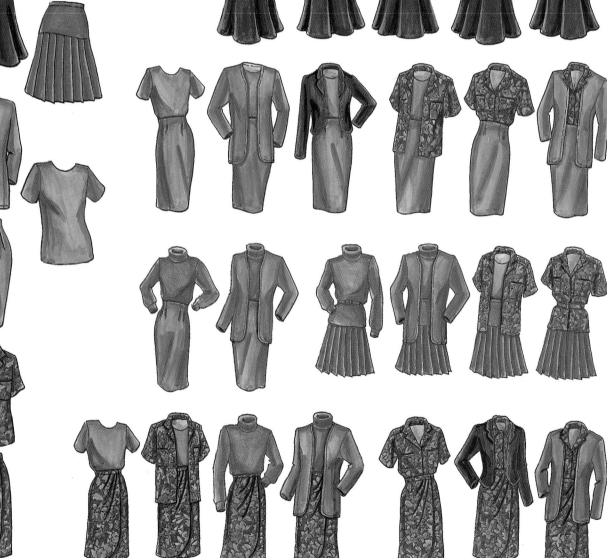

Connecting Capsules

If you plan carefully, pieces from the second capsule can link with pieces from the first to form a new capsule of their own—a wardrobe that really WORKS!

Start With...

- red jacket and skirt from the first capsule

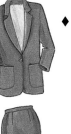

- navy jacket and skirt from the second capsule

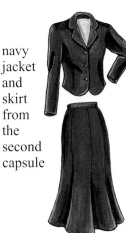

Then Add...

- white blouse
- yellow turtleneck
- nautical scarf

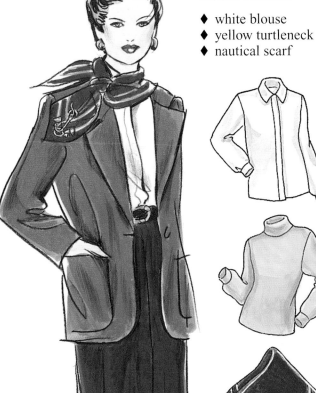

Start With...

- royal jacket and skirt from the first capsule

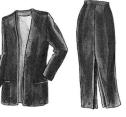

- black pants from the first capsule
- black turtleneck from the first capsule

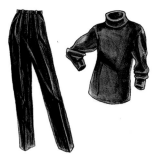

Then Add...

- jade/royal scarf
- black/jade/fuchsia scarf

- jade jacket, skirt and shell from the second capsule
- fuchsia turtleneck from the second capsule

ADRIENNE VITTADINI

Casual Capsules

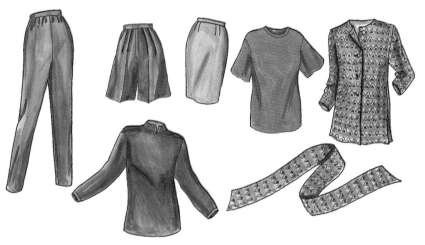

The capsule concept is also a life-saver in the most challenging wardrobe situations. For example, many of us spend so much attention to our career or public wardrobes that we dress like rag-bags at home.

A capsule of mix-and-match sportswear can remedy the situation. Consider cotton-blend knits for comfort and easy care. They are cool in summer and can be layered for cozy warmth in winter, so choose seasonless colors for year-round wear.

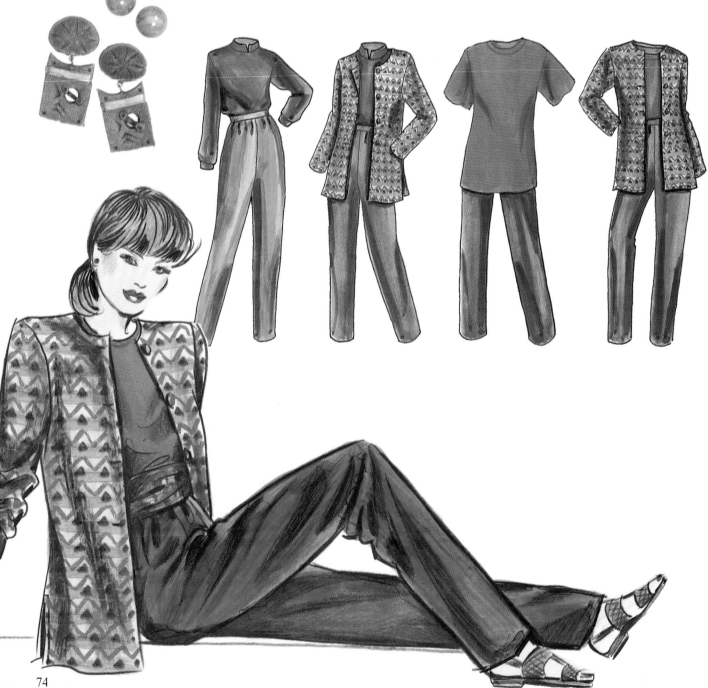

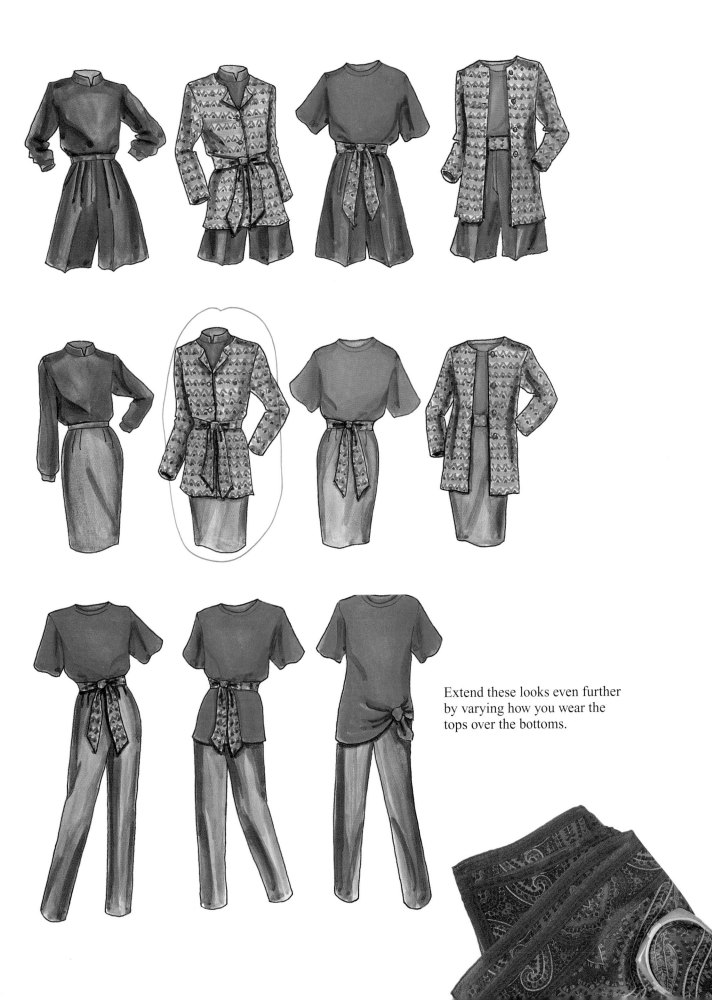

Extend these looks even further by varying how you wear the tops over the bottoms.

If knits aren't your style, here's an
alternative casual capsule of denims,
woven cottons and T-shirts,
with warm and cool
color suggestions:

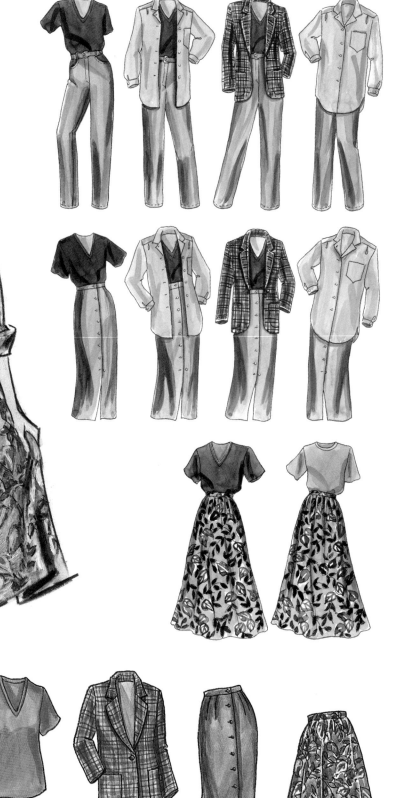

Cool Colors

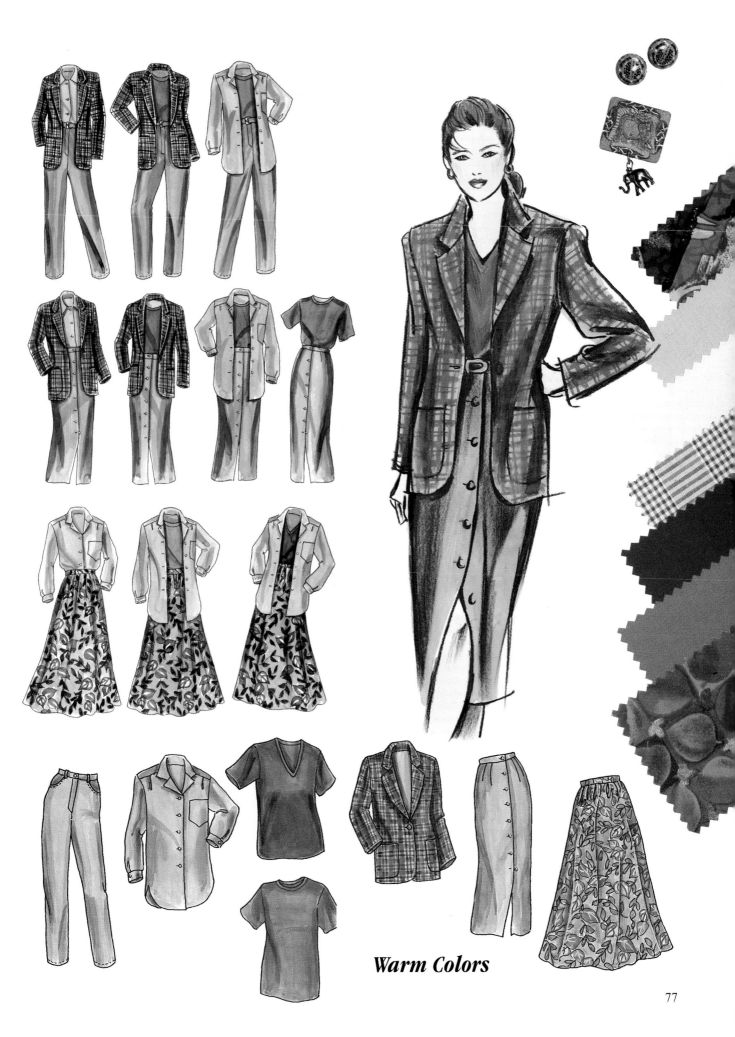

Warm Colors

Evening Capsules

Dressy social occasions are a major wardrobe challenge for most women. We love to look special, but hate to spend big money for a knockout, wear-it-once garment. (See cost per wearing formula, page 119.)

Capsuling is the answer again. A carefully selected group of separates can take you through a decade of dressy affairs without anyone thinking "She wore that last year."

Choose late-day fabrics, such as silks or silkies, crepe de Chine, silk jersey, silk crepe, velvet, satin and metallics.

Add a new item or two each year and you'll never regard a special invitation as a closet crisis again.

Tailor the exact choices to your personal style, but follow this basic format.

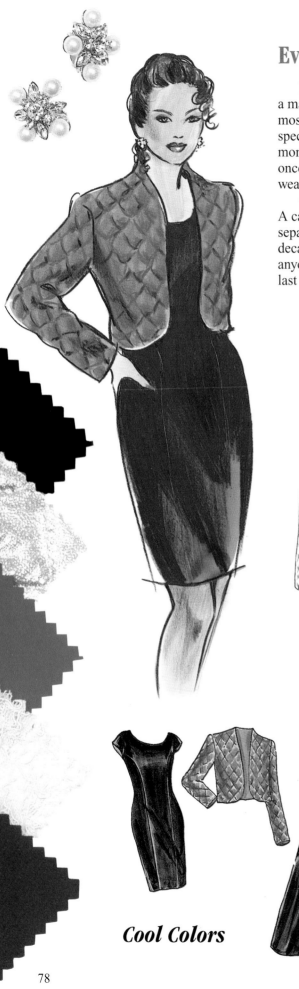

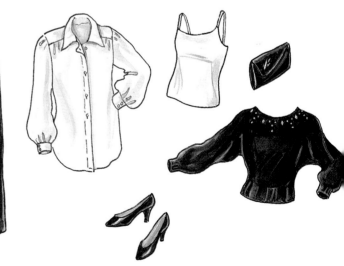

Cool Colors

Dress for not-quite-so-formal occasions by mixing your evening capsule items with pieces from your regular wardrobe. For example: The camisole and earrings can dress up a collarless wool crepe suit for a cocktail party. The quilted jacket can top gabardine trousers and a silky shell for a holiday open house.

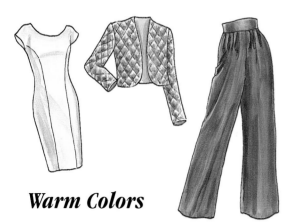

Warm Colors

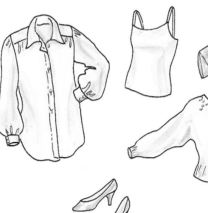

Creative Capsuling

Capsuling is a very practical approach to wardrobe planning. Now here are some ways to add your own personal pizzazz and make that practical wardrobe exciting too.

Fashion Personality

Our sample capsules were fairly Classic, but if your fashion personality is more Sporty Natural, High-fashion Dramatic or Feminine Romantic, you can easily add those self-expressive touches with accent pieces or with accessory choices.

Try adding a white blouse, another sweater and coordinating accessories to your basic capsule, choosing designs that match your personal style.

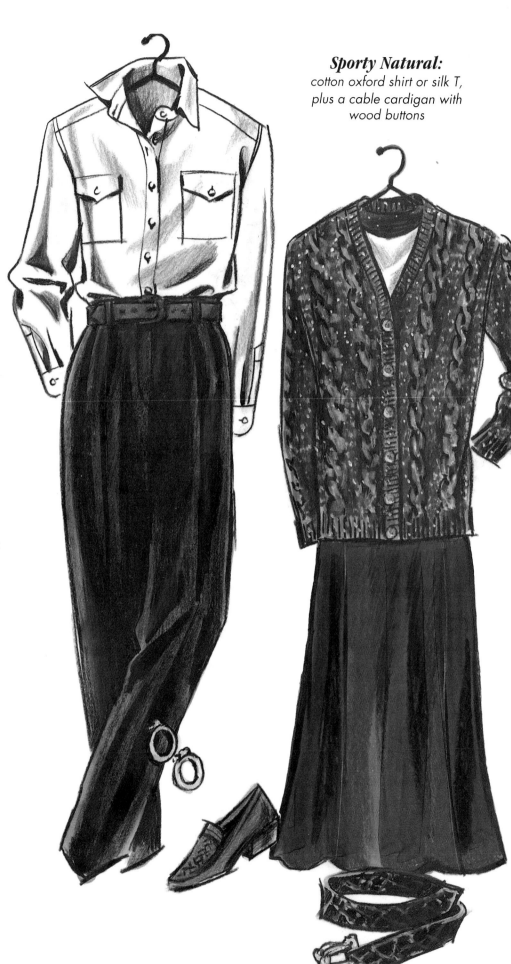

Sporty Natural:
cotton oxford shirt or silk T, plus a cable cardigan with wood buttons

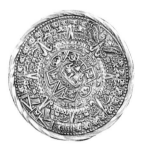

High Fashion Dramatic:
asymmetrical blouse with draped lapel
and a sweater with dramatic geometrics

Feminine Romantic:
blouse with soft ruffles and
lace and a short, fitted-waist
sweater with openwork
yoke and pearl
buttons

81

Mix Textures

Designers like Calvin Klein and Bill Blass use unexpected texture contrasts to add classic individuality. Mixing textures is easier than mixing patterns. Here are some guidelines:

1. Medium textures are easiest to work with. They combine well with each other and with other smooth or highly textured surfaces.

   ♦ Flannel trousers mix easily with a satin blouse and sweater-knit jacket.

2. Unless you want the truly unexpected combinations of sequins and denim, or suede and satin, combine extreme textures only if they are similar in mood.

   ♦ Mix sequins with satin; mix suede with wool tweed.

Mix Prints

Mix prints, or prints and plaids? Of course!

♦ Men do it daily when they combine subtly patterned suits, shirts and ties.

♦ Designers like Missoni and Koos Vanden Aker built international reputations on it.

♦ Patchwork quilts raise print mixing to an art form.

You will get the best mix of patterns when you tie them together with either color or design.

♦ If the colors are different, the design shapes should be similar.

♦ If the print designs are different, they should be in closely related colors.

♦ Vary the scale. If one print has large shapes, the second should have smaller shapes. A third could be a coordinating stripe.

The easiest combinations are meant-to-match prints.

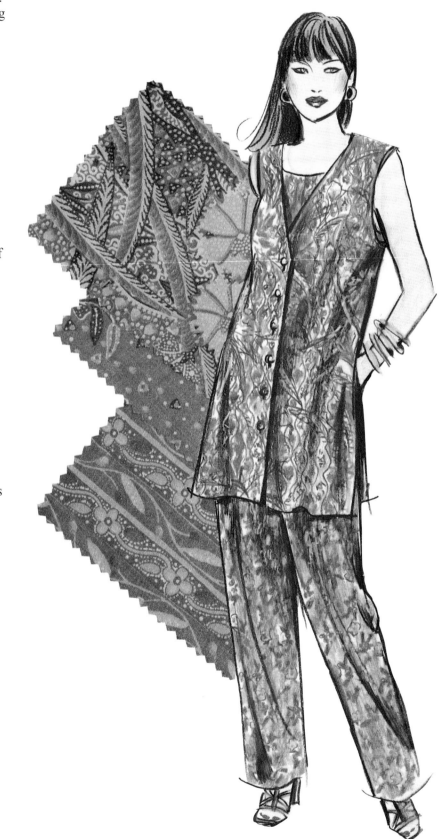

Try a mixture of plaids in similar colorations and varied sizes.

The blouse-weight print repeats the colors from the wool plaid.

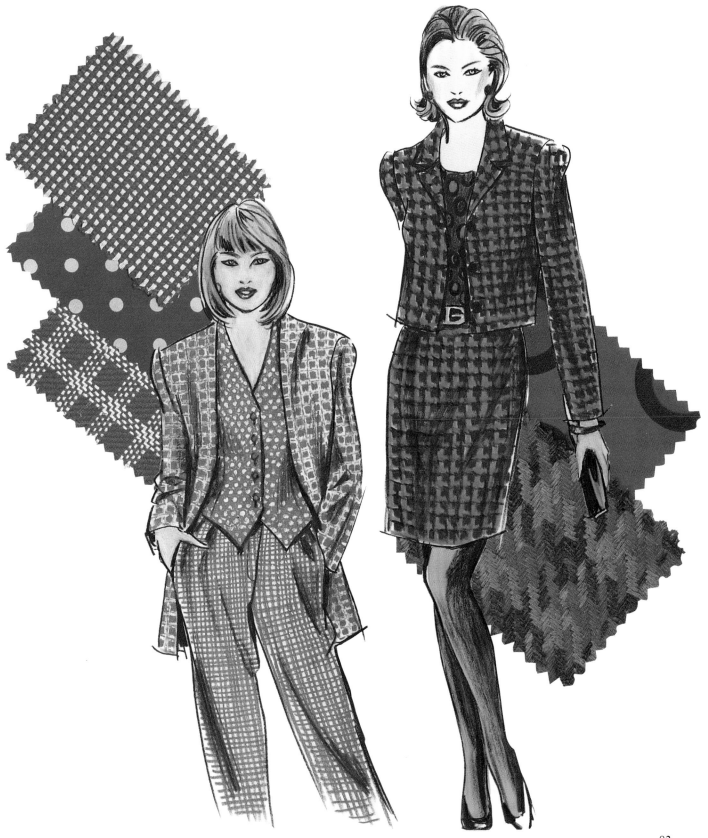

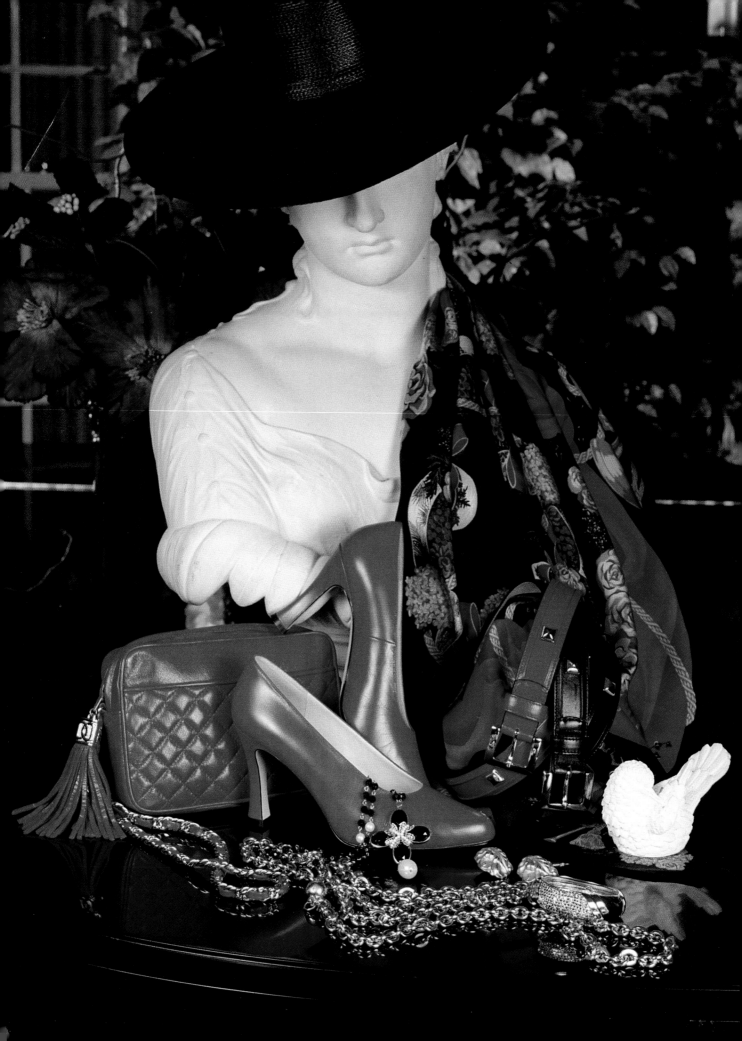

CHAPTER 6

Accessory Impact

The Accessory Advantage

Accessories can be the glue that holds your wardrobe together, linking separate garments into fashion-right ensembles.

They are great wardrobe extenders because they create the illusion that you are wearing a different outfit every day.

Top wardrobe consultants often guide clients to spend as much as a third of their wardrobe budget on accessories. They are a wise investment because they last years longer than most garments.

And they aren't affected by your weight and size variations either. Did you ever hear anyone say "I've gained weight and can't squeeze into my earrings"?

So invest in the best accessories you can afford. Good pieces in classic designs are always in style. It is better to avoid spending on faddish pieces that are just "throw away chic."

Then use your accessories to:

♦ Revive or update wardrobe classics and old stand-bys.

♦ Change an outfit instantly from a daytime look to after-five.

♦ Add color and life to neutral garments.

♦ Focus attention exactly where you want it.

Shoes & Hose

Footwear must be comfortable. You can't present an appealing look when your face is grimacing in pain.

Leather is the best investment for comfort and durability. Shop in the middle of the day—feet are smallest in the morning and often swollen in the evening.

Considering the cost of better leather goods, your selections should work with most everything in your wardrobe. Shop with your color swatch palette and keep your personal style in mind.

Best Bets to Buy

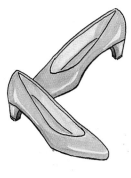

1. If you can afford only one good shoe, make it a closed-toe pump in black or taupe (cool) or beige (warm). These seasonless neutral colors will blend with everything, and a pump can work with both skirts and pants.

2. Shoe color should be the same value or darker than your hemline to ground the look and avoid calling attention to the feet.

3. A 1½ - 2" heel is flattering to most legs. Wear a minimum of 1" heel if you are heavy, short or short-legged.

4. The lower the top of the shoe and the more instep that shows, the longer your legs look. Avoid T-strap styles unless you can afford to make your legs look shorter and heavier.

5. The more foot that shows, the less businesslike the shoe. Strappy, sling-back sandals are clearly dressy shoes. However, a simple closed-toe, sling-back pump can be a comfortable alternative for business occasions.

6. Keep your shoes in top repair. Have new heel tips put on as soon as the original ones begin to show wear. Touch up tiny nicks in the leather with a color-matched permanent marker.

Boots

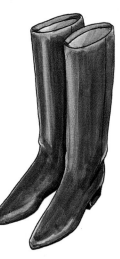

In colder climates simple, classic boot styles in quality leather are a good investment. Neutral colors are best. A classic black boot is easy to dress up or down. Burgundy is another good choice that blends with both black and brown clothing. Make sure there is no gap between the top of your boot and your hemline.

Choose additional shoes based on your lifestyle and your personal style. The chart below presents some options.

	Evening	Casual	Sports
Tailored Classic	peau silk pump with gold trim	tassled walker	sneakers
Feminine Romantic	strappy sandal	bowed ballet flat	sneakers
High-Fashion Dramatic	jeweled 3" heel	patchwork metallic slip-on	sneakers
Sporty Natural	plain peau	penny loafers pump	sneakers

Hosiery

You look instantly taller and trimmer when you match the color tone of your hosiery to your shoe and your hem.

1. With a neutral-colored skirt or pants, match all three color elements. Example: black skirt, off-black hose, black shoes.

   This concept works well with neutrals like navy, gray, brown, beige, taupe and even burgundy and rust, but NOT with red.

   Colored hosiery for dressy or business situations should be very sheer. Charcoal gray or off-black is more subtle than a solid black.

2. With a brightly colored garment, choose neutral shoes and match hose to shoes. Example: red dress, taupe hose and taupe shoes.

3. Two-color spectator pumps look best with hose matched to the lighter color, NOT the darker one.

4. Very dark, light or bright hosiery colors and patterns or textures draw attention to your legs.

5. Off-white or light beige can be worn with black during the summer season.

6. Keep leg coverings in the same mood and weight as your shoes. Chunky, casual shoes work with heavier, textured hose or socks.

7. Avoid emergencies by purchasing hose in quantity and keeping a spare pair in your desk drawer and/or automobile glove compartment.

Belts & Bags

Belt Basics

♦ Leather belts in widths from ¾" to 1½" are fashion classics worth collecting in a variety of your best colors.

♦ Belts that match or blend with the color of your garment are less eye-catching and give the illusion of a longer body line.

♦ Contrasting belts add more visual interest, an extra plus if your waistline is a figure asset.

♦ A bold decorative buckle draws attention to the center of the body and visually slims the figure. The effect is even more pronounced when the belt is worn under an open jacket.

♦ Wider belts are more comfortable in soft materials. They also work best on a figure with a long torso and not too much waistline shaping.

♦ Matching a belt to your blouse color can elongate a short-waisted figure. Matching the belt color to skirt or pants can minimize a long-waisted silhouette.

♦ Look for best belt buys on sale. Shoe repair shops can inexpensively reposition the buckle on a too-long bargain belt. They can also recycle a favorite buckle from an old belt and attach it to a new one.

Bag Basics

You "wear" your handbag every day, so it makes sense to invest in a good one. That investment can be sizable, so think basic in both color and style.

♦ It is no longer a rule that your bag must match your shoes, but matching bag color to the shoes you wear most often does simplify things.

♦ Neutral colors are the best investments
COOL - black, taupe, gray, navy,
         cordovan (a brown-burgundy)
WARM - brown, camel, rust, beige, warm gray

♦ Leather is the best choice for year-round use. In warm weather, neutral-colored canvas or straw work with any shoe color.

♦ Make sure the bag you're considering will hold your normal contents. Empty the purse you are carrying into the new one to check its capacity before your buy.

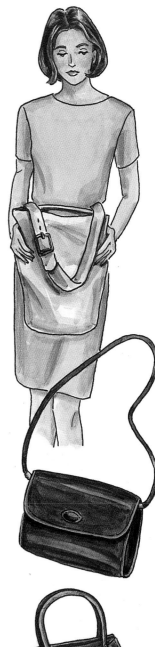

♦ Try on a purse before you buy to be sure it compliments your body proportions. If it is larger than the area between your waist and hips it is probably too big for you.

♦ A shoulder bag is convenient. Be sure the strap is short enough for the bag to hang at the top of your hipbone. Hanging it lower will add width to your silhouette. A shoe repair shop can shorten a too-long strap.

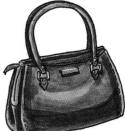

♦ The handbag style is another classic. If the straps are long enough, the bag can be worn over the shoulder for added convenience and safety.

♦ Envelopes and clutches are a dressier look, ideal for business women to slip into a briefcase.

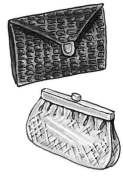

♦ The best evening investment is a small clutch in black or metallic.

Briefcases

- Choose a briefcase in quality leather that matches or blends with the color of shoes you wear most often. Darker leathers look more expensive. Cordovan (a brown-burgundy) is a versatile choice.

- A leather tote is a less formal alternative to the briefcase, great for more relaxed career looks.

- A softer portfolio shape is more feminine than the traditional structured style.

- Consider owning two briefcases—one of quality leather for fall/winter and a lighter-colored canvas or straw for warm-weather months.

Look for practical details such as:

- Detachable shoulder strap for easier carrying when hands are full.

- Double stitching, reinforced handles and metal corners for durability and long wear.

- Inside compartments for easy organization.

- Sturdy clasps or top zipper for security.

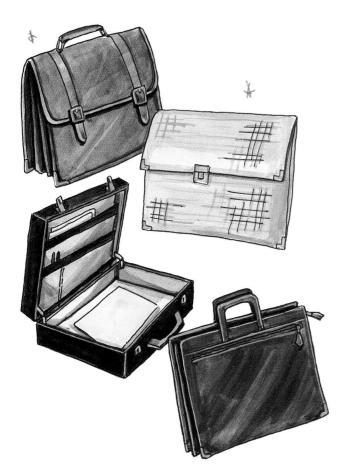

Scarf Savvy

Scarves are a surefire way to pull together unrelated separates. Update a dress or blouse in a less-than-best shade by using a scarf to frame your face with a flattering color.

Scarves instantly draw attention upward on your body, creating a taller, trimmer appearance.

Keep these points in mind when you shop:

- Oblong scarves are the most versatile.

- Multicolor print scarves that combine several of your best colors are the best investment. The style of the print should relate to your personal style (Romantic florals, Dramatic abstracts, etc.).

- Silk scarves tie easily and drape beautifully. Only the finest polyesters even approach silk's beauty.

- Wool and rayon challis scarves look great in cool weather, but can be bulky to tie. Drape them over a shoulder instead.

- Economical cotton bandanas can add pizzazz to very casual sportswear for just pennies.

- Straight-grain scarves tie crisper bows; bias-cut scarves fall more softly.

- Good scarves never go out of style, so invest in scarves you love and wear them for years.

- Try folding larger square scarves into versatile oblong shapes like this:

wide to narrow oblong   *square to triangle*

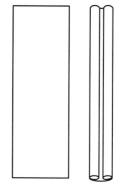

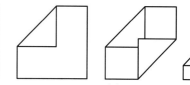

square to oblong

Tie One On

Entire books are written about "50 Nifty Ways to Tie a Scarf"...but this versatile favorite works six different ways and isn't tied at all.

You'll need:

♦ A rectangular scarf (or large square folded diagonally to a triangle).

♦ A tiny rubber band or 1/2" plastic curtain ring.

1. Drape the scarf around your neck with the ends hanging evenly in front.

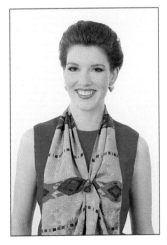

2. At about bustline level, tuck a little bit of each scarf edge through the rubber band or ring.

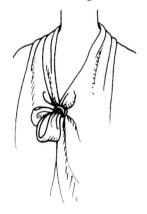

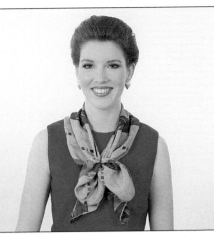

Look #1 - *Gradually pull through more and more fabric to form a mock bow.*

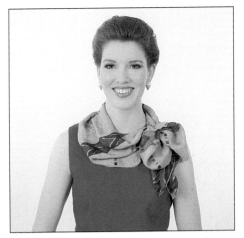

Look #2 - *Rotate the scarf around your neck, bringing the bow to the shoulder. Secure it with a fine silk pin or a bit of double-stick fabric tape.*

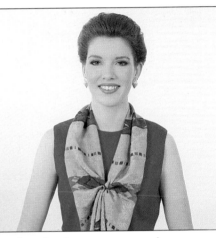

Look #3 - *For variety, use the same technique EXCEPT pull the scarf edges through the rubber band toward the inside—next to your body. The result is a softly draped jabot.*

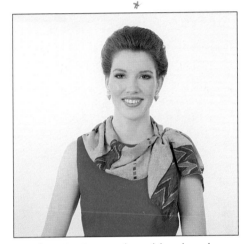

Look #4 - *Rotate the rubber band to the shoulder, draping one scarf tail to the front and the other to the back.*

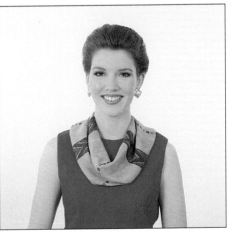

Look #5 - *Rotate the rubber band to the back. The front forms a graceful cowl. Tuck the tails into the back neckline of your blouse or jacket.*

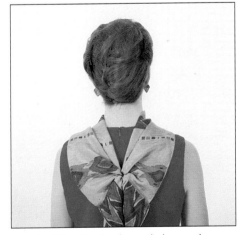

Look #6 - *Or let the tails hang down the back for a fashion-forward look.*

More Easy Scarf Techniques

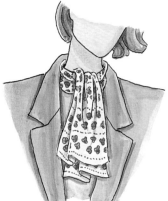

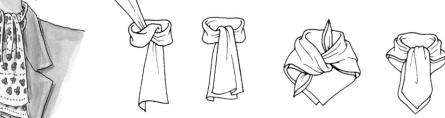

Try the classic ascot from an oblong scarf or a folded square.

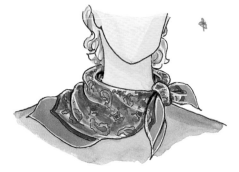

A new angle on the cowboy scarf—tie a square knot (remember Girl Scouts—right over left, left over right) and shift the knot to front, back or side.

Fill in an empty neckline for a soft splash of color.

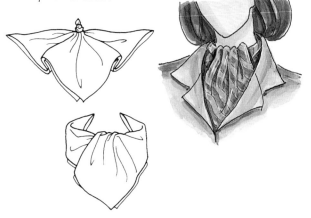

Frame your face with a centered knot, then tie at the back.

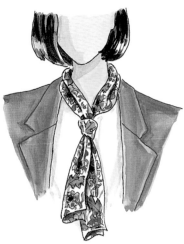

Turn a scarf into a "necktie"...

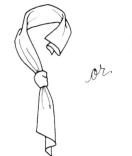 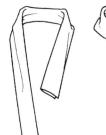 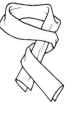 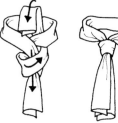

Add dash with the "flip"...

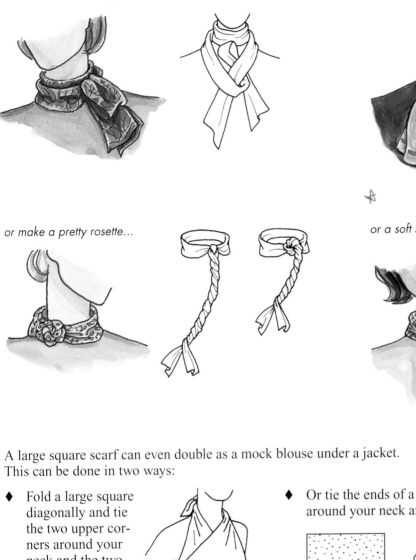

or loop the loop...

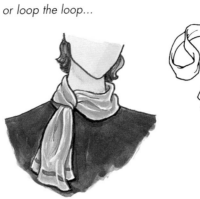

or make a pretty rosette...

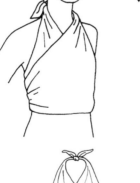

or a soft stock tie.

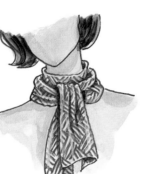

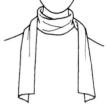

A large square scarf can even double as a mock blouse under a jacket.
This can be done in two ways:

♦ Fold a large square diagonally and tie the two upper corners around your neck and the two lower corners around your waist.

♦ Or tie the ends of a large square around your neck and waist.

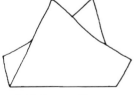

fold diagonally

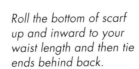

Roll the bottom of scarf up and inward to your waist length and then tie ends behind back.

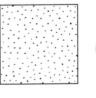

Jewelry

Jewelry is the accessory element with the greatest potential for creativity and self-expression. Jewelry choices fall into three basic categories:

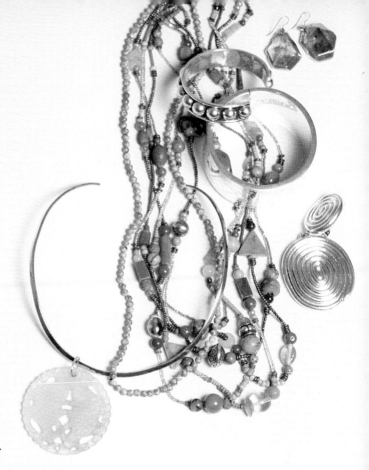

- ◆ **Fine jewelry**—precious metals and gemstones have a timeless appeal, but few of us can afford an extensive wardrobe or statement fashion pieces in this price category.

- ◆ **Bridge jewelry**—items made from semi-precious stones, shell, natural woods, enamels and porcelains give a lasting, quality look at reasonable prices. This category usually offers the best investments for your jewelry wardrobe.

These natural materials have the added advantage of blending with a wider range of garment colors than their plastic copies. Choose items to compliment your coloring and wardrobe:

Amethyst, for example, will blend with a wide range of lilac, lavender and purple shades because of its own variegated color.

Paua and *abalone shell* absorb the colors around them, so they work well with nearly any shade of blue, green, purple, beige or gray.

Turquoise and *jade* can enhance eye color.

Carnelian, jasper, amber and *wood items* are versatile choices for a warm-toned wardrobe, accenting brown, beiges and rust.

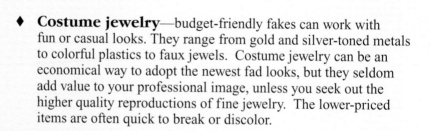

- ◆ **Costume jewelry**—budget-friendly fakes can work with fun or casual looks. They range from gold and silver-toned metals to colorful plastics to faux jewels. Costume jewelry can be an economical way to adopt the newest fad looks, but they seldom add value to your professional image, unless you seek out the higher quality reproductions of fine jewelry. The lower-priced items are often quick to break or discolor.

♦ Use jewelry to create visual illusions, balance your proportions and direct the viewer's eye to your assets.

Bold earrings draw attention instantly to your face—and if the material relates to your eye color the effect is even stronger. Abalone or paua shell is an especially flattering choice for people with blue/green/gray eyes.

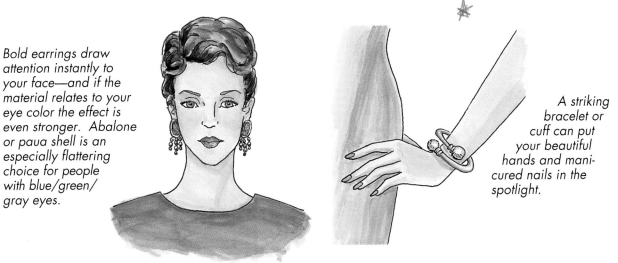

A striking bracelet or cuff can put your beautiful hands and manicured nails in the spotlight.

♦ Create the illusion of an ideal facial shape.

Round earrings and choker-style necklaces add needed width to a long, narrow face.

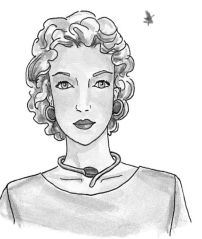

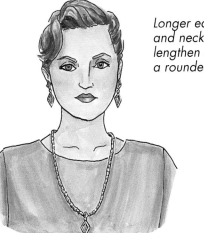

Longer earring shapes and necklaces can lengthen and narrow a rounded face.

♦ Balance body proportions.

A bold pin, placed fairly wide on the shoulder, diverts attention away from broad hips.

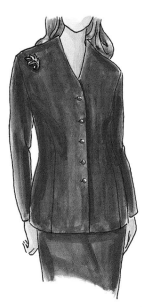

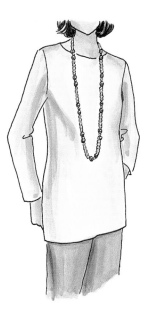

A long necklace worn with a tunic creates the illusion of a longer-waisted figure.

Spend Your Jewelry Dollar Wisely

Try on jewelry items before you buy. Make selections based on how the pieces look on you, not just their intrinsic beauty or how well they match a particular garment.

Color—use your color swatch palette to help you select jewelry that will enhance your coloring and work with many items in your wardrobe.

Which metal? Remember the gold/silver test for determining your cool or warm undertones? (See page 23.) If one metal looked decidedly better on you, it should be your preference for jewelry. If both metals seemed flattering, you can choose gold or silver accessories.

Even if the silver looked best, you can still wear gold in a less brassy tone and in small amounts. If the gold looked best, you should also consider accessories in brass, copper, or a combination of gold/silver/copper.

If you wear both gold and silver, a few pieces that combine both metals in one design will help you coordinate your jewelry wardrobe more easily. A watch that combines both metals is especially versatile.

Jewelry Guidelines

Wear your jewelry and accessories with panache, using the guidelines that follow.

Metals range in tone from warm coppers and brass to both warm and cooler golds and the cool silvers. Some pieces of jewelry combine metals, making them a versatile addition to your wardrobe.

♦ Bottoms Up! When your top and bottom garments are different colors, create visual unity by repeating the bottom color in jewelry items. We show turquoise earrings and button covers here.

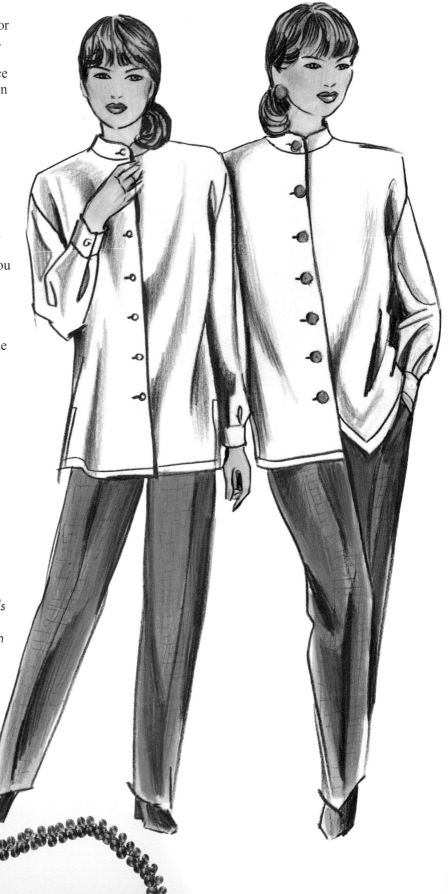

94

♦ Repeat one color. When accessorizing a print or plaid garment, keep all the accessory accents in the same color. We've used black as the unifying element below. A red, white and blue plaid accessorized with red earrings, white necklace and blue bracelet would look spotty and out of harmony.

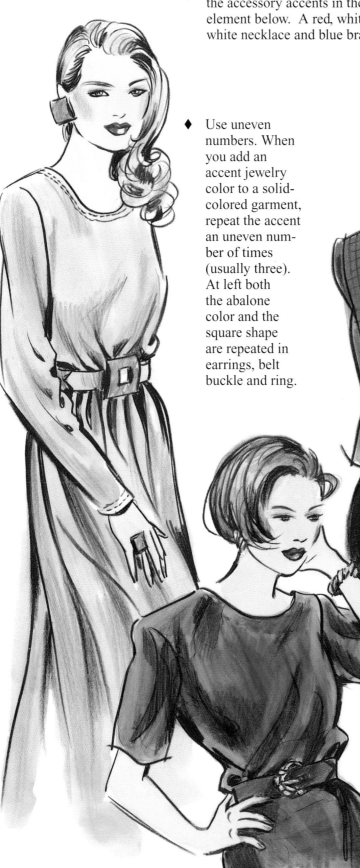

♦ Use uneven numbers. When you add an accent jewelry color to a solid-colored garment, repeat the accent an uneven number of times (usually three). At left both the abalone color and the square shape are repeated in earrings, belt buckle and ring.

♦ Repeat your metal. If one jewelry item has a bold metallic accent, repeat that metal at least once more in the ensemble for visual unity.

Accessories help basic clothes adapt to the mood of an occasion, or to your Personal Style.
See how the same garment can become...

Classic   **Natural**   **Romantic**   **Dramatic**

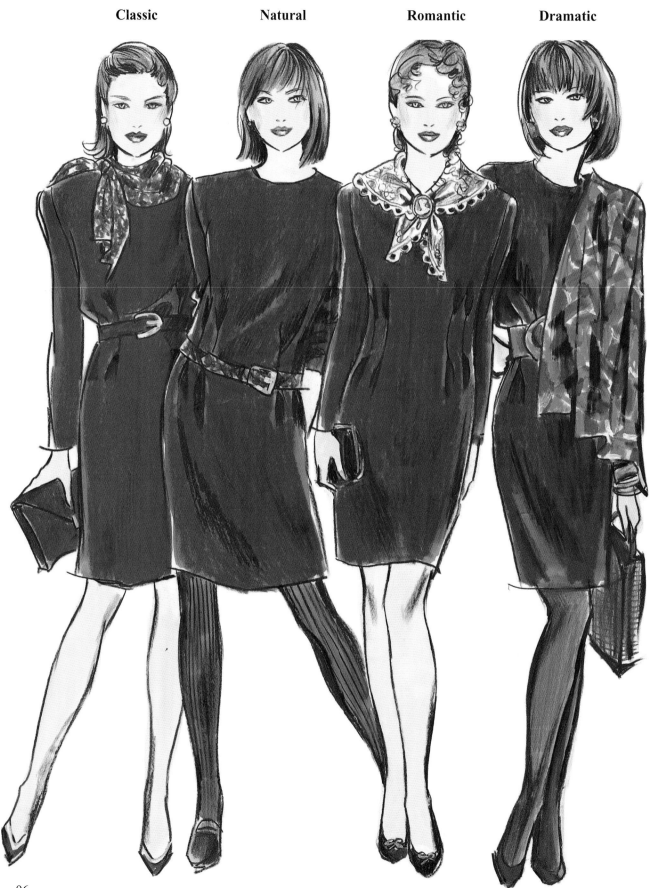

Build Jewelry "Capsules"

You've already learned to get more versatility by planning your garments in coordinating groups.

The same concept applies to jewelry. Select several pieces that work well together. If your best metal is gold, select a number of good, basic gold items—a chain, basic stud earings, a larger pair of gold earrings, and a gold bracelet. For dressier occasions, add a simple string of pearls, then a pair of pearl earrings. Over time, collect items to create jewelry capsules that make a statement about you and your own personal style.

Use your creativity to find multiple ways to wear your capsule items:

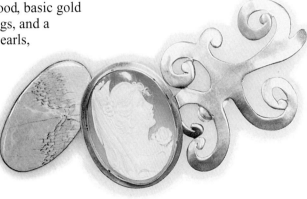

A pin on your lapel is just the beginning...

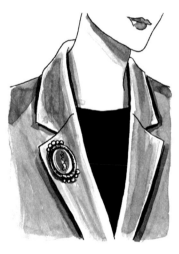

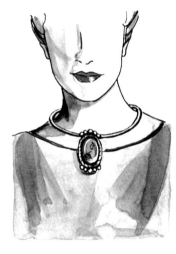

Hang it from a metal neck wire.

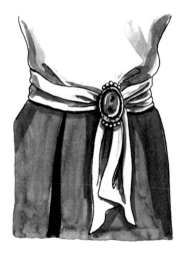

Pin it onto a sash like a belt buckle.

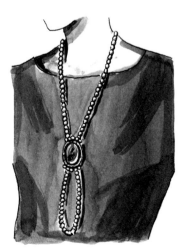

Pin it across a strand of beads, bolo style.

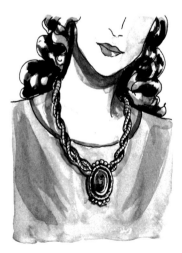

Twist two strands of beads and secure them with a pin.

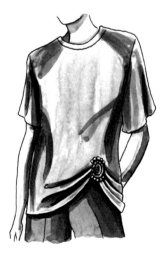

Gather up the hem of a T for a flattering diagonal.

Multiple uses for a slide-style belt buckle.

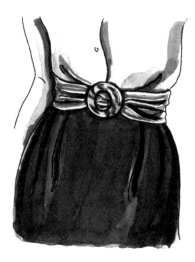

Use it as a buckle with a fabric sash

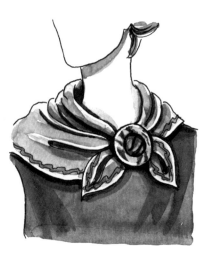

...as a dramatic scarf holder.

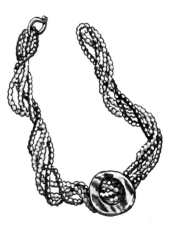

...as a pendant on twisted strands of beads.

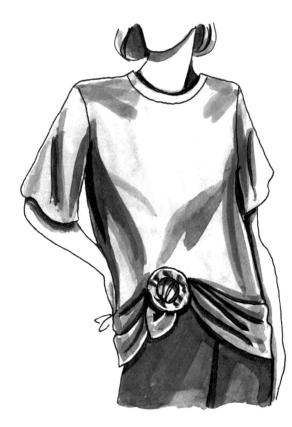

Gather the edge of an oversized T.

Give basic earrings added pizzazz.

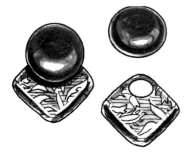

Add a metal jacket or enhancer behind the earring.

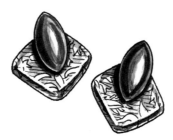

Another day, wear the same jacket with a different type of earring.

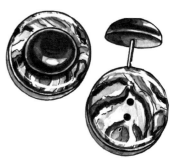

A great button can become an earring enhancer if the holes are near the middle!

Make a necklace the right length for your garment neckline.

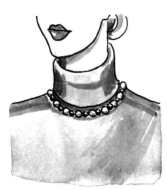

Too short?

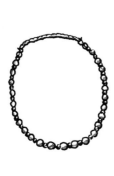

Hook in a plain bracelet to extend the length.

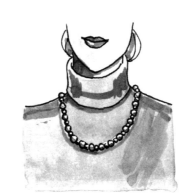

Just right.

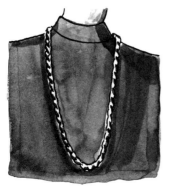

Too long?

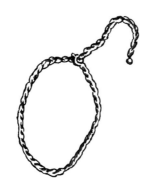

Hook the clasp closer in along the strand.

Create the stacked Chanel look.

Create the stacked Chanel look easily with one or two long strands wrapped several times around your neck.

Arrange the loops so they fall gracefully. Try this with gold chains, pearls, or a combination.

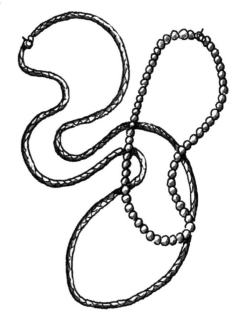

99

Look Better Proportioned... INSTANTLY!

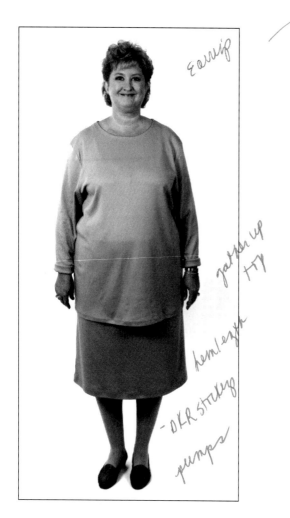

A perfectly good garment can still be all wrong...without the right accessories and details.

Here we have added shoulder pads and a diagonal hip treatment to this two-piece knit dress. The skirt has been shortened to a more flattering length and tapered to create a slimmer look. (Not an accessory item, but what a difference! See page 147 for how-tos.) Brighter makeup and bolder earrings draw the attention to the face. A more flattering leg line is created with low-heeled shoes and hose that blends with them.

These accessory concepts can be combined to trim visual pounds from your figure.

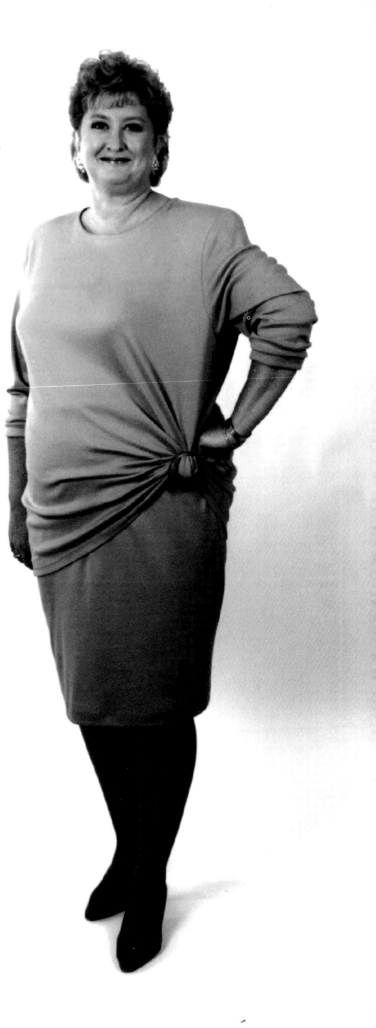

Don't Ruin Your Image

The smallest details can make or break the look you've worked so hard to create.
Guard against these typical troublemakers.

Problem:	*Solution:*
Rundown shoes	Work with a good shoe repair person; use a felt marker to touch up scuffs; put a piece of soft carpet under your feet when you drive.
Reinforced-toe nylons with open-toe shoes	Buy sheer-toe nylons and strengthen the toe seam with liquid seam sealant before wearing.
Nylons with runs	Keep a spare pair in your car glove box or desk drawer.
Underarm stains	Prevent them with dress shields.
Lint or dandruff	Keep a small lint brush in car/desk.
Missing/loose buttons, snaps, hooks	If you can't repair them yourself, ask your dry cleaner.
Slips that show	Own several in assorted lengths.
Slipping lingerie straps	Notions departments sell tiny strap holders you can sew into the shoulder seam of any blouse.
Visible bra/panty lines	Substitute panty hose to eliminate lines; be sure bras are properly fitted; check rear view in full-length mirror.
Linings hanging too long	You or a dry cleaner can fix this easily.
Too-short coat over longer shirt	Buy your coats extra-long with this issue in mind; they are warmer that way.
Too-tight pants; slim skirts	If body-shaping undergarments won't solve the problem, alter the garment or retire it.
Blouses gapping at bustline	If a better bra doesn't help, don't wear the garment.
Garments with pilling, fading or stains	Carefully remove pills with a defuzz gadget or a razor; try bleach on stubborn stains and consider dyeing a faded item.
Unkempt or outdated hair	Work with a hair pro to find a style that fits YOUR hair texture and styling ability.
Roots	Touch-ups can be expensive, so consider highlighting instead of allover color.
Unmanicured/chipped nails	New quick-dry polishes and top-coats make manicures and touch-ups quick and long-lasting.

And ALWAYS, ALWAYS check your total look—front and back—in a full-length mirror before you leave the house. Far better for you to see a problem first than for others to see it all day.

Accessory Add-Up

Fashion consultants often use a point system to be sure a look is neither overdone nor boring.

Give yourself one point for each of the following...and an extra point for any item that is especially bold or ornate:

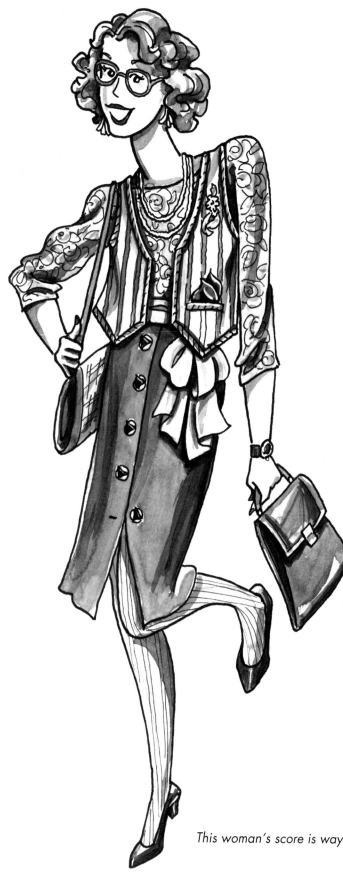

___Each visible item of clothing

___Each accent color

___Each patterned/textured fabric

___Each decorative trim

___Each piece of jewelry

___Colored nail polish

___Colored or textured hose

___Handbag

___Briefcase

___Contrasting belt

___Scarf or pocket hankie

___Decorative buttons

___Eyeglasses

___Hose that blend with shoes

___Low-heeled (not flat) shoes

___ **Total**

If your total falls below eight you probably need to add an accent or two to avoid looking bland.

If you score over 14 you are probably overdressed. Remove or change something to create a more pleasing, unified appearance.

This woman's score is way over 14!

CHAPTER 7

About Face

Mastering Makeup

Even the most spectacular wardrobe can't create your best appearance if your face is either unfinished or overdone.

Far too many women skip makeup entirely because they want a "natural look." But the truth is that well-done makeup looks more natural than your bare face...and naturally gorgeous at that.

The key to effective makeup lies in selecting colors that blend with your own coloring while emphasizing and enhancing it. Your color swatch palette is a good guideline.

♦ Foundation should match your skin tone as exactly as possible.

♦ Eye shadow colors should include:
—A base color that blends with your skin tone
—An accent color that relates to your hair color
—A second accent that either repeats or complements your eye color

♦ Blush and lip colors should blend with the pink/red or peach shades from your swatches.

♦ Eye liner and mascara relate to your seasonal classification. Cool seasons can choose dark brown, gray or navy; warm seasons look best in warm brown tones. Few women can look natural wearing black liner.

When you choose makeup colors this way, they will blend with everything in your wardrobe. You won't need special makeup colors for each outfit. How beautifully simple!

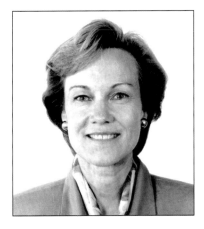

Without makeup a woman might look tired. The complimenting colors of correct makeup can energize her appearance. This woman is our "Spring" model on page 25. In the photo of her on that page you can study her makeup in color. Turn to page 106 to see her in both casual and glamour makeup.

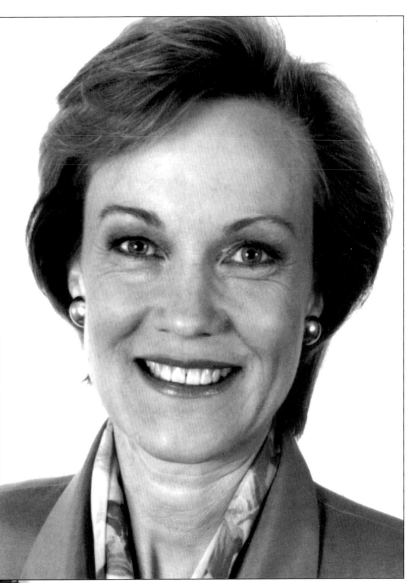

The 10-Minute Face

Styles in makeup application change over time, but with these instructions you can complete a timeless classic look in less than 10 minutes.

On the grid below dab samples of your colors, recording their names in the boxes at right.

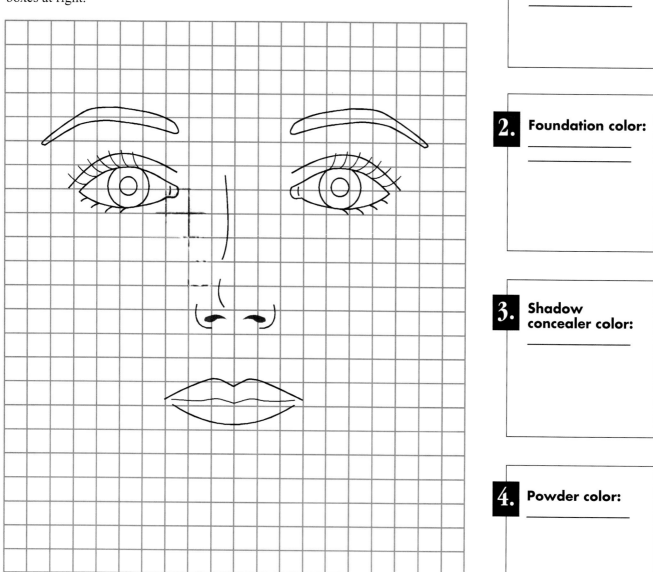

Evaluate the finished makeup job in a full-length mirror. You should see your facial features more distinctly, but scarcely notice the makeup itself.

Don't be surprised if your first trial of our "10-Minute Face" takes a little longer. With a few days of practice, you'll soon reach an efficient pace.

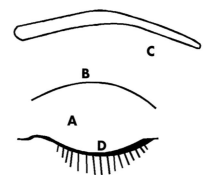

1. **Color-correction cream colors:**

_____
_____
_____

2. **Foundation color:**

_____
_____

3. **Shadow concealer color:**

_____

4. **Powder color:**

_____

5. **Eye shadow colors:**

A. _____
B. _____
C. _____
D. _____

Step 1: Conceal any unwanted coloration in your facial skin with a color-correction cream.

These creams rely on basic color theory: blend a color with its complement (color wheel opposite) and it disappears.

♦ Conceal ruddiness with mint green

♦ Conceal a sallow, yellowish cast with lilac or blue-pink

♦ Conceal blue-purple veins with yellow

Dot the cream on the colored areas with a cotton swab. Blend the color with a makeup sponge until it looks slightly chalky.

Step 2: Even out skin tone with a light layer of foundation.

Pour a bit of the liquid onto a makeup sponge. Dot some onto your forehead, cheeks, nose and chin. Blend it over your entire face, using downward strokes with the sponge.

Step 3: Conceal dark circles.

Nearly everyone has slightly darker coloration just below the eyes, giving the effect of dark circles if it isn't lightened with a cream concealer. Dot the concealer on with a cotton swab. Carry it up to the lash line, but down no farther than the bone. Blend with a sponge.

Step 4: Dust on a light coating of a finely milled powder.

Powder sets the foundation and gives the skin a velvety look. Try powdering only one side of your face and look at the difference!

Step 5: Eye shadow isn't a mystery.

Start by applying a pale shade over the entire lid, from lashes to brows, from inside corner to outside corner. This should be barely visible, since the color blends with your skin. Accent the crease with a small area of the second color just above the iris and under the brow bone. Add color accent and visual spacing with a third color at the outer corner.

Use a sponge to blend the accent shades until their color is subtle. Finish with a soft pencil liner right along the lash line. Line from the outer corner about halfway in on top, about 1/3 of the way in on the bottom. Blend the liner with a cotton swab (or the cap of the liner pencil) to smudge and soften the look.

Step 6: Add a light coat of mascara.

Let it dry, then add a second coat for more fullness. Mascara is a fertile growth medium for bacteria; replace it every 90 days. Rinse and keep the old applicators, though. They are great for combing through any clumps that form on your lashes.

Step 7: Brows form a natural frame for your face.

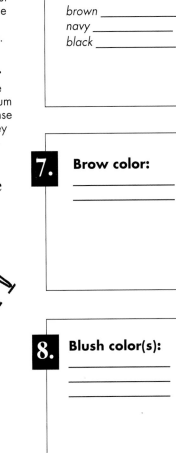

Define yours with a soft pencil or powdered brow color, following your natural shape. Bushy brows look more controlled and skimpy brows gain fullness from a brow styling gel. Brush it through the brows, then style them into a lifted shape.

NOTE: If you need to tweeze your brows, coat them first with baby teething gel to numb the "ouch."

Step 8: Apply blush with a soft brush.

Start at the hairline and come toward the center of the face along the top of the cheekbone. That higher placement visually lifts the face and adds sparkle to the eyes. Use a clean brush to blend the edges of the blush for a softer, natural look.

Step 9: Lip liner gives a crisply defined mouth shape.

Sketch a generous line of color outlining the top and bottom lips. To make lips appear fuller, line along the ridge of skin where the lip structure begins. To minimize full lips, line just inside the ridge, where the natural lip color starts. Add tiny fill-in strokes of liner and blend with a fingertip. This added liner maintains some color on the lips long after lipstick has worn away.

Step 10: Lipstick adds polish to your look.

At the same time, its emollient ingredients keeps lips moist and conditioned. Use a lip brush for an even, precise application and greater staying power.

6. Mascara colors:

brown _____
navy _____
black _____

7. Brow color:

_____
_____

8. Blush color(s):

_____
_____
_____

9. Lip liner color:

_____

10. Lipstick colors:

_____
_____
_____
_____

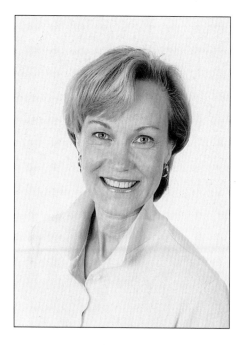 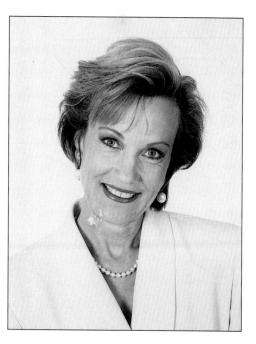

Casual Face

Glamour Face

For sports or very casual occasions, a lighter makeup look is best.

For glamorous evenings, jewel-tone makeup colors and more dramatic applications are ideal.

♦ Apply foundation with a slightly damp sponge for more sheer coverage.

♦ Use more vivid eye shadow accent colors; eye liner is definitely noticeable. Brow color should be more prominent and lashes need several coats of mascara.

♦ Eliminate accent eye shadow colors; use only base color and pencil liner. Keep mascara application light.

♦ Keep lip colors natural and glossy.

♦ Apply lip liner to the outer edges for the fullest look. Lipstick colors should be bright and glossy or frosted.

♦ A generous application of a pale blush adds a healthy glow.

♦ Use a brighter blush, but a very sheer application, so focus goes to eyes and lips.

Skin Care Basics

Healthy skin is critical to a good makeup application...and to a positive, attractive image. A good skin- care program can significantly retard the inevitable aging process.

Lifestyle factors are as important as creams and lotions in caring for the skin. Skin is, after all, a body organ—by far the largest, in fact—so all the factors that contribute to overall health also help develop glowing skin.

♦ Getting adequate sleep gives the skin cells down time to produce new cell layers.

♦ Consuming six to eight glasses of water daily hydrates the skin from within, and flushes away the by-products of cellular reproduction.

♦ Eating a healthful diet provides the nutritional building blocks for new tissue growth.

♦ Avoiding caffeine and nicotine prevents constricted (tightened) blood vessels. When the blood flows freely, it carries nutrients to the developing skin cells.

♦ Avoiding sun exposure prevents ultraviolet rays from damaging the connective tissue in the skin's supporting layer. Dermatologists call sun exposure the single greatest cause of premature aging and wrinkling.

Getting Better With the Years

Aging doesn't have to result in the stereotype of sagging, wrinkled skin. We CAN get better as we get older! In the photos here, you see a range of ages in several women who look better today than ever. Stay out of the sun and heed the skin care advice below to maintain your own good looks for years to come. And update your hairstyle and wardrobe regularly with the strategies presented in this book—and you'll gain more self-confidence and polish at the same time.

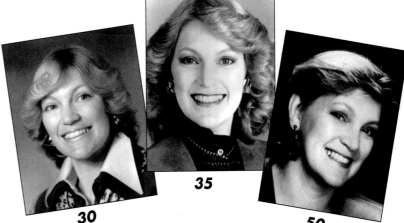

30   35   50

A woman can continue to look good... or even better... as the years pass by.

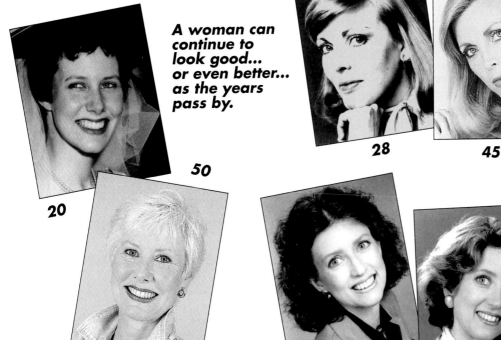

20   50   28   45   55

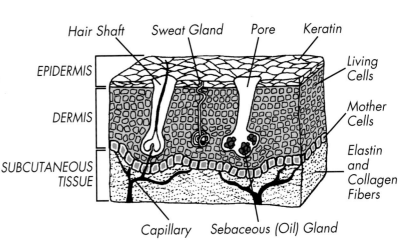

35   40   45

Understanding how skin grows helps clarify the need for proper skin care. New cells are produced in the innermost layer and are gradually pushed toward the top by yet newer cells as they form.

This migration takes about 21 days, and by the time a cell reaches the surface, it has lost most of its natural moisture and plumpness. Eventually these aged cells are sloughed off.

The under layer, the dermis, nourishes and supports the outer layer. It contains blood vessels to feed developing cells and elastin and collagen to keep skin firm. It includes sweat glands and sebaceous glands that empty oil and perspiration through the pores.

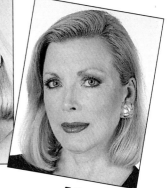

Hair Shaft   Sweat Gland   Pore   Keratin

EPIDERMIS

Living Cells

DERMIS

Mother Cells

SUBCUTANEOUS TISSUE

Elastin and Collagen Fibers

Capillary   Sebaceous (Oil) Gland

Daily Skin Care

Effective skin care can take just moments each morning and night. It consists of:

♦ Cleansing to remove surface debris and keep pores from becoming clogged,

♦ Exfoliating to remove dead surface cells, and

♦ Moisturizing to keep the skin supple. Regardless of the brand of skin care you select, it is important to use a compatible group of products. Each line is formulated so all components work together for optimal results. Mixing brands can sometimes create unexpected reactions.

Cleansing

A facial cleanser lifts away makeup, oil, perspiration and pollutants without stripping the skin of needed moisture or leaving a residue.

Apply cleanser to the face with an upward/outward motion and massage gently. Rinse with a soft washcloth and tepid water.

Some skin care systems include a toner or astringent to re-establish the skin's normal pH balance. Apply the liquid to a cotton ball and stroke it over the skin.

Other cleansers are themselves pH balanced and don't require a companion toner.

Exfoliating

Exfoliating removes dead cells from the skin's surface so the younger, fresher ones beneath are visible. This can be done manually, using a product with a gritty texture that literally scrubs away the outer layer of cells.

Or it can be accomplished chemically instead. A relatively new classification of ingredients called alpha-hydroxy acids breaks down the chemical bonds between dead skin cells, perspiration and body oils, so the debris rinses away without scrubbing.

Moisturizing

Moisturizers protect the skin against drying, keep it soft and supple, and minimize wrinkling. A light film of moisturizer in the morning helps makeup go on smoothly and serves as a buffer against pollutants in the air.

A richer night-time moisturizer nourishes the skin during its rejuvenating process.

Women with oilier skin need an oil-free moisturizer applied sparingly.

Facial Shape

The shape of your face is an important element of body style. If you've been confused in the past about which of those dozens of facial shapes matches yours...relax.

Pull the hair back from your face and stand in front of a mirror. Use the corner of a bar of soap to draw on the mirror an outline of your face.

Notice whether your face is long and narrow, short and wide, or the ideal balanced proportion.

It is easy to balance a disproportional facial shape with flattering choices in hairstyles, necklines and accessories.

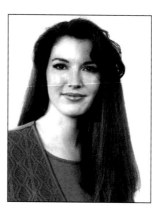

Give a better balance by changing the hair style to flatter the shape of the face.

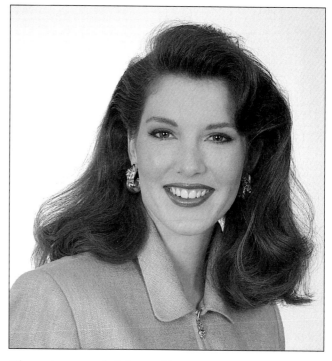

Elongate a rounded face with:

♦ a narrow, lifted hairstyle

♦ open V necklines

♦ earrings that are longer than their width

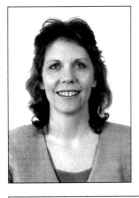

Add a flattering width to a narrow face with:

- a fuller hairstyle; forehead-concealing bangs
- higher, rounded necklines
- choker-style necklaces
- wide or rounded earring shapes

Also decide in front of a mirror whether your jaw line and facial features are more angular (think of Cher or Barbra Streisand) or more softly rounded (like Rosie O'Donnell or Oprah Winfrey).

Angular faces look most harmonious with hairstyles, accessories and clothing details that are similarly angular.

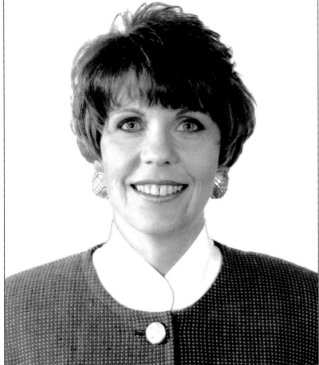

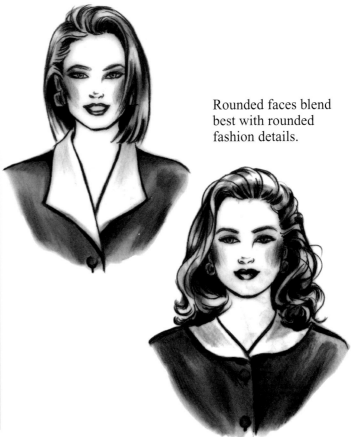

Rounded faces blend best with rounded fashion details.

Wearing Glasses

You can make a spectacle of yourself the right way by selecting frames that complement your skin tones, eye and hair colors. Gold or tortoise-shell frames look terrific on women with warm coloring. Women with cool undertones look better in silver or subtly marbleized blue or wine.

If you have only one pair of glasses, don't color-coordinate glasses with garments. Frames should enhance your facial features, not accent your clothes. If you want to make a color-cordinated fashion statement, buy an extra pair to have fun with.

Gear your eye makeup to your glasses. A prescription for farsightedness will magnify the eyes—and any accompanying makeup. So apply subtle colors with a light touch and balance the look with bright lip color. On the other hand, a prescription for nearsightedness will minimize eyes. Counter with bolder eye makeup and softer lip color.

Hair Color

That woman whose hair color you admire just may be chemically enhancing it. The obvious dye jobs you spot from across the street are the ones that don't work. Here are some tips to ensure that a hair color change looks natural:

1. Don't make a radical change from your natural color. One or two shades lighter or darker are usually the best choices.

2. Stay within your seasonal color range. Red hair on a cool-skinned person almost always looks artificial. And it constantly surrounds her face with a color she would never select in clothing.

3. For a lighter color with less maintenance, try streaking some strands near your face several shades lighter than your overall color.

4. Professional hair color products vary in their coverage, from translucent to opaque. Ask for a sheer wash of color, rather than a heavy opaque one, so that the natural light/dark variation of your hair shows through.

5. Test a new color you're considering via a wash-out color rinse, a wig or the new computerized imaging process.

Working With Your Stylist

Don't be too intimidated to tell even the most celebrated stylist what you want in a haircut. Her expertise plus your communications can add up to the style of your dreams.

The stylist needs to know:

♦ How much money you're willing to spend on maintenance cuts,

♦ Whether you have the time and expertise for blow drying, special brush techniques, etc.,

♦ Special demands of your career,

♦ The kind of clothing you usually wear,

♦ Any body challenges you want your haircut to minimize,

♦ Past haircuts you loved, or hated.

Hairstyle

Hairstyle is a very visible component of your total image...and often a challenging one. Even a recent Miss America referred to having the infamous "bad hair days."

It is worth almost any investment of time and money to find a stylist who can create a look that's right for:

♦ your facial shape
♦ the nature of your hair
♦ your personal style
♦ your career needs

A change in hairstyle can add or diminish fullness in your facial shape, creating the illusion of the fashion-ideal oval.

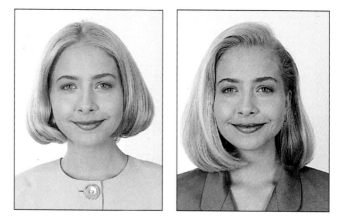

Texture

Fine hair gains bulk from a blunt cut no more than chin length. Substitute tapering for layering if you want a softer look around the face. Body-building shampoos and setting lotions add volume, but their slight residue means you'll need to shampoo more frequently.

Medium hair is easiest to handle. Blunt cuts create a bulkier look than angled cuts, which make hair lie closer to the head. Layered cuts add fullness.

Coarse hair can look bushy if not carefully styled. Avoid volume-enhancing blunt cuts. Moderate length adds some control to coarse hair. Or go very short and let it curl. Use a softening conditioner and skip setting lotions.

Be cautious about straightening very curly hair. The harsh chemicals, if overused, can leave hair looking like straw.

Personal Hairstyle Categories

Various styles also express the four
personal style categories.

Dramatic

Natural

Classic

Many career fields demand hairstyles that are conservative and neat. If your career needs run counter to
your personal style, find a hairdo that can be worn
more than one way.

Romantic

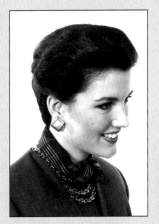

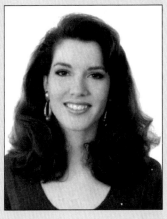

CHAPTER 8

Before You Shop

Become "Fashion Fluent"

To win at wardrobe planning, learn to adapt what's in fashion to your personal needs. That means selecting a balance of classics, current fashion trends and an occasional fad.

The Fashion Curve

The direction in which fashion evolves can be plotted like this:

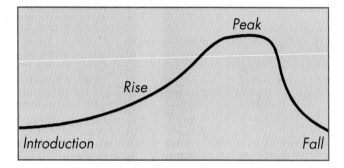

Introduction—a fashion trend is usually introduced by a high-fashion designer who creates expensive one-of-a-kind styles, often too extreme for the average person.

Rise—the designer look is copied for mass production by high-quality manufacturers. The style is modified to lower prices, but the item is still expensive and somewhat extreme.

Peak—additional modifications have been made to lower the price and make the style more moderate for acceptance.

Fall—there is so much of the look that everyone who wants it has it. It goes on clearance-sale racks and the manufacturer stops making it. This fall happens very quickly compared to the rise.

NOTE: As mass communications have spread fashion news and connected people world wide, there seems to be less fashion "dictation." However, there will always be some trends. Will skirt lengths and pant leg widths always offer the variety we have today?

Timing Your Purchases

Any item at its peak is one you won't be able to wear for long. One just beginning to rise is a better buy. In other words, if you buy the style that everyone is wearing now, it will likely be out of fashion before you've gotten your money's worth of wear from it.

Sometimes we just don't get around to adding a new look as soon as we intended, and it's already past its peak. Or we spot a look we like, but realize it's just a fad. If you must add it to your wardrobe, accept the fact that you will probably wear it for only six months or so and plan your expenditure accordingly.

Fads and Classics

Both fads and classics have their special place on the fashion curve.

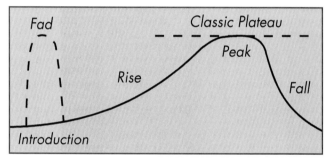

Fads are short-lived styles. They rise very quickly to their peak, then fall with equal speed. Fads are often characterized by:

♦ Gimmicky details like nonfunctional pockets or buttons.

♦ Bright, loud colors like chartreuse or iridescent orange.

♦ Glaring prints using bold colors and high-contrast combinations.

♦ Exaggerated details like very wide, curiously shaped collars.

Classics are no-nonsense pieces that withstand influence from trends and fads. They are usually designed with simple, clean lines that allow you to adapt them to continuing style changes. Classics are the old reliables...never so "in" this season that they'll be "out" next year. They give you even more for your money when they are made from high-quality fabrics and neutral colors.

Classic Styles:

Shirtwaist dress	Turtleneck
Cardigan jacket	Convertible-collar blouse
Blazer	Bow blouse
Shawl-collar blazer	Crew & V pullover sweaters
Chanel jacket	Cardigan sweater
Slim, fitted skirt	Trousers
Dirndl skirt	Jeans

Classic Details:

Set-in sleeves	Medium-width collars, lapels
Hems near the knee	Medium-width sleeves

Do Your Fashion Homework

Early each season, "snoop shop" to get ideas for what new color stories and design details are being featured. Looking is FREE...and FUN.

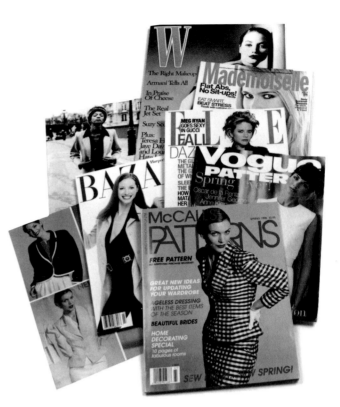

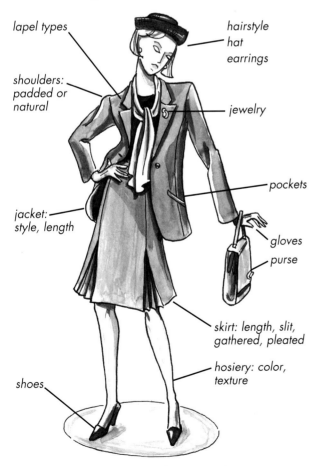

lapel types

hairstyle
hat
earrings

shoulders:
padded or
natural

jewelry

jacket:
style, length

pockets

gloves

purse

skirt: length, slit,
gathered, pleated

hosiery: color,
texture

shoes

Study In-Store Fashion Displays

Magazines

Get an overview by reading fashion magazines—both editorial features and fashion ads. Vogue, Harper's Bazaar, Mademoiselle and Glamour are good choices. Also consider "W," a bimonthly condensation of the fashion news that appears in Women's Wear Daily, a trade publication for buyers and designers.

Remember that much of what magazines feature is the most extreme example of what's to come. By the time it reaches the majority of stores, it will be toned down to appeal to the average consumer.

Read a magazine by flipping through the pages checking only ONE detail at a time. Check only hemlines, perhaps, then page through again noting only shoulder lines and sleeve styles. Next time through, focus on collars or whatever.

Pay special attention to accessories and how they are worn. And notice hairstyles shown with newer fashions. A dramatic clothing change often requires a change in hairstyle to balance the look.

Budget

Image consultant Susan Bixler estimates the average American woman wastes 55 percent of every clothing dollar on ill-advised purchases. If that's correct, vowing to spend wisely—whether your budget is large or small—is equal to a half-price savings on everything you select.

Avoid costly impulse purchases by planning your wardrobe and your budget in advance. Go through the last 12 months of your check registers and charge account statements and add all wardrobe expenditures. The total may surprise you.

Next apply cost estimates to the items on your needs list from your Wardrobe Work Sheet (pages 62-63). Generous estimates are better than conservative ones. They help prevent buying poor quality items just for their lower prices. And you'll feel great if you find some true bargains and have some budgeted funds left over for wardrobe extras.

Remember to budget for accessories too. Many wardrobe consultants advise clients to spend as much as one-third of their money for shoes, belts, scarves and jewelry pieces to finish outfits with polish and pizzazz. Accessories provide an instant update for older garments. And they last longer than most garments, so they need replacing infrequently.

Plan your payment methods carefully. You can spread one shopping trip's purchases over several months' budgets by using a combination of cash or checks, charge cards and lay-away.

If your budget simply won't finance your planned purchases, decide which items can wait. Better to purchase some things at end-of-season sales than to settle for lesser-quality pieces that will look shoddy and wear out quickly.

A Fashion Dictionary

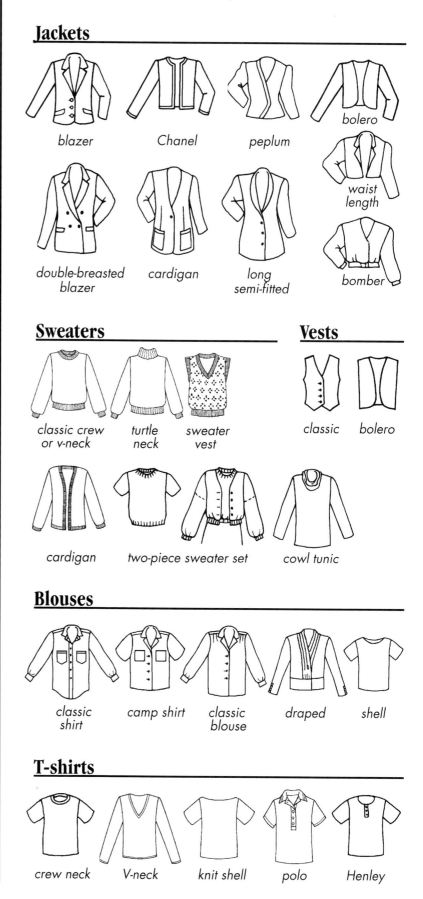

Jackets

blazer

Chanel

peplum

bolero

double-breasted blazer

cardigan

long semi-fitted

waist length

bomber

Sweaters

classic crew or v-neck

turtle neck

sweater vest

cardigan

two-piece sweater set

cowl tunic

Vests

classic

bolero

Blouses

classic shirt

camp shirt

classic blouse

draped

shell

T-shirts

crew neck

V-neck

knit shell

polo

Henley

Skirts

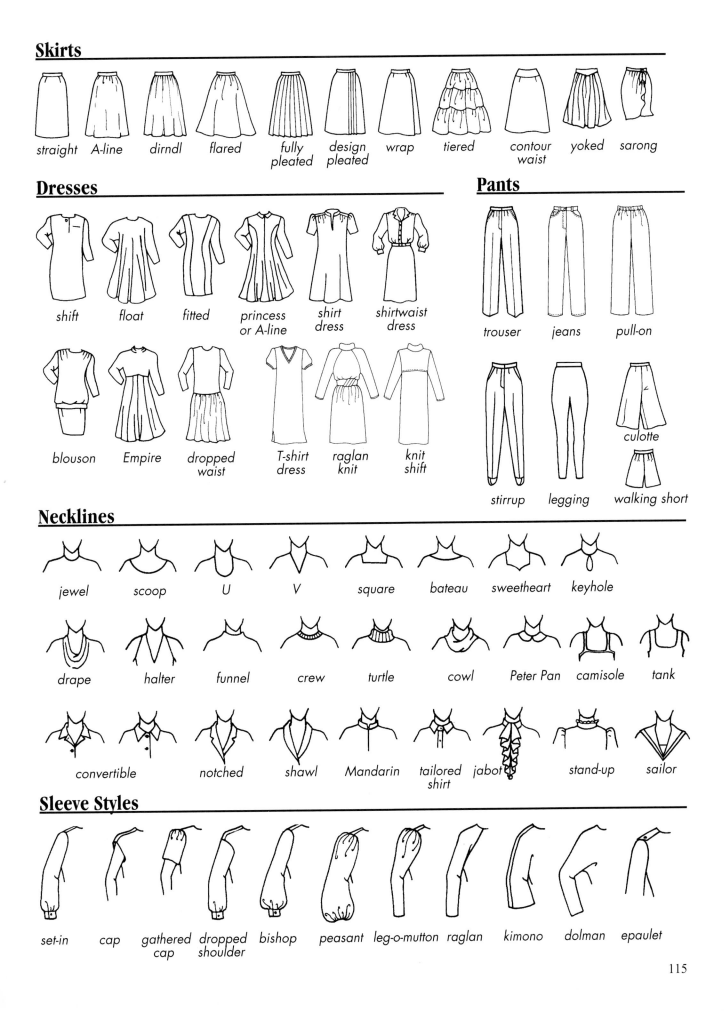

straight A-line dirndl flared fully pleated design pleated wrap tiered contour waist yoked sarong

Dresses

shift float fitted princess or A-line shirt dress shirtwaist dress

blouson Empire dropped waist T-shirt dress raglan knit knit shift

Pants

trouser jeans pull-on

stirrup legging culotte walking short

Necklines

jewel scoop U V square bateau sweetheart keyhole

drape halter funnel crew turtle cowl Peter Pan camisole tank

convertible notched shawl Mandarin tailored shirt jabot stand-up sailor

Sleeve Styles

set-in cap gathered cap dropped shoulder bishop peasant leg-o-mutton raglan kimono dolman epaulet

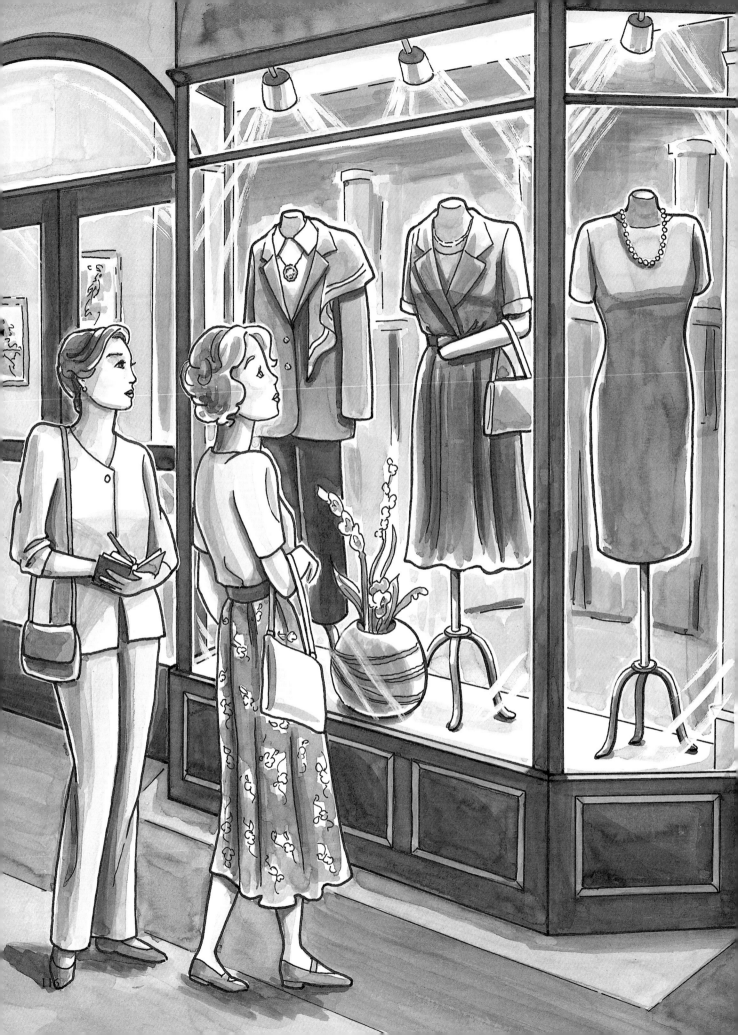

CHAPTER 9

Shopping Smart

Snoop Shopping

Snoop shopping means looking in better stores for things you've seen in magazines, but leaving your money at home.

First just browse, paying particular attention to:

♦ Window displays and mannequins

♦ How new looks are accessorized

♦ What makes something look "now" instead of last year

You can and should try on anything that catches your eye. Don't let price tags discourage you. You didn't bring any money anyway!

Try experimenting with colors and styles that don't appeal to you. You already know how you look in your usual styles, but there might be some equally flattering new ones you've never tried. Critically evaluate what you see by standing as far as possible from the mirror to get the full effect.

♦ Do the design lines accentuate your assets or your figure challenges?

♦ How does the fabric look, feel and move on your body?

♦ Is the color good on you?

♦ Does it fit within the range of your personal style?

Take notes on what you liked (and didn't), but DON'T BUY ANYTHING. Go home and rest up for a serious shopping expedition another day.

Shopping Smart

On Shopping Day, dress in good underwear, comfortable shoes and easy-off clothing. Be sure to bring:

♦ Your seasonal color swatches

♦ Your swatch file of current clothes

♦ A Need list, copied from the Wardrobe Work Sheet you created during your closet clean-out and capsule planning session (page 63)

♦ Items you plan to match, but couldn't swatch

♦ Dressier shoes for trying on dressier clothes

"Bottoms-Up" Shopping

Plan to buy the very best quality items you can afford. But you don't have to pay the most money for them. From the information in this chapter you will learn to recognize quality, regardless of the price tag.

So if your budget is tight, organize your shopping expedition by the "Bottoms Up" method. That means starting at the lowest-priced stores first and working up to department stores and boutiques, if necessary.

Consider These Choices:

♦ Department stores and women's specialty stores are the top of the shopping ladder for selection and amenities. For bargains, plan your shopping around the store's special promotions. (Apply for a store charge and you'll get advance notice of sales.)

Go to the store the night before the sale. Sometimes you can buy at the special price then. But if not, you still have a chance to browse, try on and make your choices in relative calm, then come back for them first thing in the morning.

You can also find bargains by shopping the boys' department. Really! Designer sportswear is regularly 25-50 percent cheaper in boys' wear than in misses sizes. Use the size conversion chart below for shirts, sweaters and jackets.

Misses-Junior	Boys
5-6	14
7-8	16
9-10	18
11-12	20

If your figure is slim-hipped, try boys' and men's pants, too. They are sized by waist and length. And alterations are usually free.

♦ Discount stores offer everyday low prices on brand-name jeans, T-shirts, sneakers, casual socks and pantyhose. Check here, too, for other sportswear, swimsuits, sandals, belts, cotton scarves and totes. Obviously, you won't find investment pieces here.

- Off-price retailers (Marshalls, Loehmans, Syms and others) and outlets do offer investment pieces, and sometimes at considerable savings.

It works this way: a manufacturer cuts 900 of a particular design. The department stores buy 800. The remaining 100 are sold to an off-price store at a reduced wholesale price or go directly to the manufacturer's own outlet store.

The store operates in a no-frills location with minimum staff to keep overhead low. Both elements of savings (low wholesale, low overhead) are passed along to you.

The selection includes broken sizes or only certain pieces of a coordinate grouping. And you have to do your own hunting, because sales people are few and far between.

But if price is the major factor in your wardrobe decisions, it pays to check the off-price retailers. Check often since new merchandise arrives weekly.

A few warnings about off-price shopping:

- Check store policies about checks, charges, returns.

- Check quality carefully since manufacturers dispose of their seconds and irregulars through these same channels.

- Be discriminating. These stores get merchandise from poor-quality manufacturers as well as fine ones. Don't get carried away by bargain prices.

- Resale shops can be a source of some almost unbelievable bargains. Seek out the ones that carry superior quality, little-worn garments. Some of the best ones are sponsored by women's civic and charitable organizations and located in affluent suburbs. Of course the selection is completely "hit-or-miss."

- Catalogs and cable-TV shopping channels are also worth considering. The big plus is convenience, since you don't even have to leave home. The catalog page or show host's description often includes details about fabric and construction quality that a typical retail salesperson might not know. Telephone-order operators can usually help you with additional questions. A minus—you can't match colors over the phone.

If you have questions about sizing, order two sizes and return the one that doesn't fit.

- Personalized trunk showings are another option to consider. Several fine-quality apparel lines are offered by independent fashion consultants across the country.

You can select the styles you like, then order them made in your size and fabric choice. Trunk shows' comprehensive color coordination makes wardrobe planning easier. Their extensive size range and custom alterations are big plusses for hard-to-fit figures. And the consultants are highly trained to recommend flattering styles and design capsule groupings.

Check the Resource List on page 155 for addresses you can contact for the name of a consultant near you.

- Sew it yourself (or have it sewn for you). If you can sew and enjoy the creative process, there's no better way of getting exactly the style, color, fit and fabric you want for your wardrobe additions... and usually at a considerable savings over designer clothing.

Chapter 12, page 133, is full of special wardrobe advice for sewing enthusiasts. To locate a skilled dressmaker, contact PACC (Professional Association of Custom Clothiers—page 155).

A Word of Caution

Don't buy any item...

- When it is about to disappear from the fashion curve.

- If it won't work with at least three other things in your wardrobe

- Just because it's on sale.

If you love sales, but fear that impulse will overrule reason...

- Shop a day or two before the sale starts and examine the merchandise at leisure.

- Make note of items that appear on your list of wardrobe needs.

- Resolve never to buy anything on sale that you wouldn't want at full price.

Cost Per Wearing Formula

To decide if a particular item is a good investment, consider its cost per wearing instead of the initial cost. Add the initial cost plus anticipated maintenance (dry cleaning, for example).

Calculate how many times you'll probably wear it. Divide the first number by the second to determine cost per wearing.

EXAMPLE: Winter coat costs $200 and will need to be dry cleaned for $25 once a year. If you wear the coat six times per week for 26 weeks a year, and keep it for two years, that totals 312 wearings.

$250 ÷ 312 = $.80 per wearing

Sequined cocktail dress on sale for $100. You can wear it to two parties this year and maybe two occasions next year.

$100 ÷ 4 = $25

The cocktail dress is a pricey choice. A capsule of dressy separates is a wiser use of your money. For evening capsule ideas, see pages 78-79.

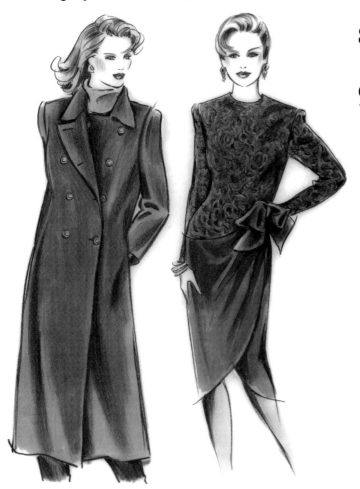

Sanity-Saving Shopping Tips

1. Shop in season, while selection is at its best.

2. Sale shoppers: Grab Need list items (pages 62-63) at the first mark-downs. Relegate that final markdown shopping trip to finding fun extras.

3. Shop when stores are least crowded— usually weekday mornings, dinnertime and in bad weather.

4. Consistently shop a few favorite stores, so sales people know you. They'll call you with word of new arrivals and impending mark-downs.

5. Don't shop at the last minute for a big event. You'll invariably buy something out of frustration that won't work well in the long run.

6. Find underwear and pantyhose you like, wait for the semi-annual sale, then stock up. You can even reorder by phone!

7. If your time is limited, shop better ready-to-wear or trunk shows. These manufacturers plan their entire line in coordinate groups to save you time putting pieces together.

8. Always shop with your colors. Don't look at anything that is not in your palette. You'll be amazed how much you'll speed your shopping.

9. Create a swatch file of current clothes to carry with you when shopping to make sure new pieces match old ones and save the hassle of possible returns. The easiest swatch file is a credit card holder filled with snips of fabric from your garments. If you sew, this is no problem. If you buy ready-to-wear, you can sometimes snip a small piece from a seam allowance...or find something else with the same color to use as your sample.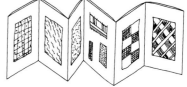

10. If you HATE to shop, have it done for you. Better stores have shopping services at no charge. Call in your list and they do the footwork for you. All you do is try on and make final selections. Free-lance personal shoppers do the same thing for a fee, and they aren't limited to one store's merchandise.

Quality Checkpoints

Always buy the best quality you can afford. It's a false economy to do otherwise, since replacements almost always cost more next year.

Here are some guidelines to help you recognize quality in garment construction, fit and fabric, regardless of the price.

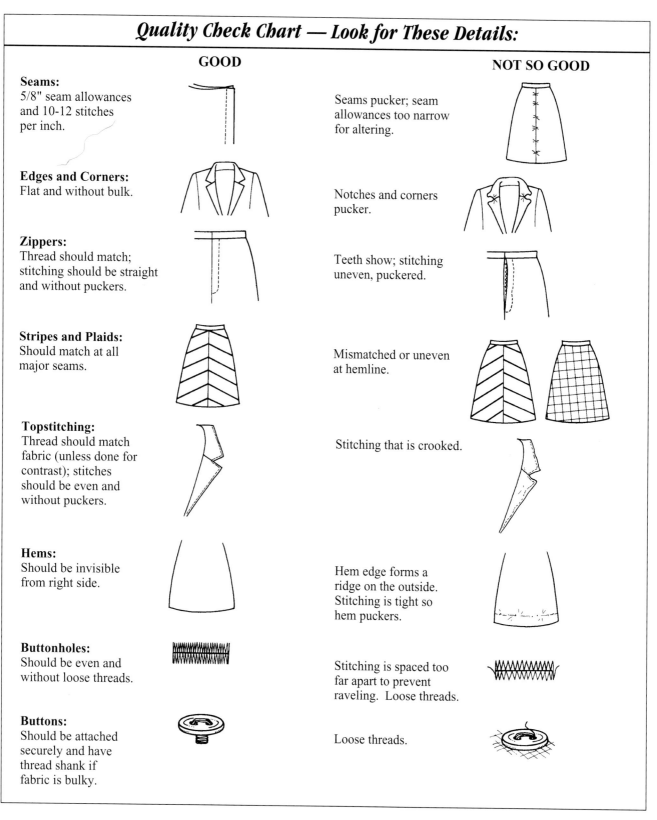

Quality Check Chart — Look for These Details:

GOOD   **NOT SO GOOD**

Seams:
5/8" seam allowances and 10-12 stitches per inch.

Seams pucker; seam allowances too narrow for altering.

Edges and Corners:
Flat and without bulk.

Notches and corners pucker.

Zippers:
Thread should match; stitching should be straight and without puckers.

Teeth show; stitching uneven, puckered.

Stripes and Plaids:
Should match at all major seams.

Mismatched or uneven at hemline.

Topstitching:
Thread should match fabric (unless done for contrast); stitches should be even and without puckers.

Stitching that is crooked.

Hems:
Should be invisible from right side.

Hem edge forms a ridge on the outside. Stitching is tight so hem puckers.

Buttonholes:
Should be even and without loose threads.

Stitching is spaced too far apart to prevent raveling. Loose threads.

Buttons:
Should be attached securely and have thread shank if fabric is bulky.

Loose threads.

What Is Good Fit?

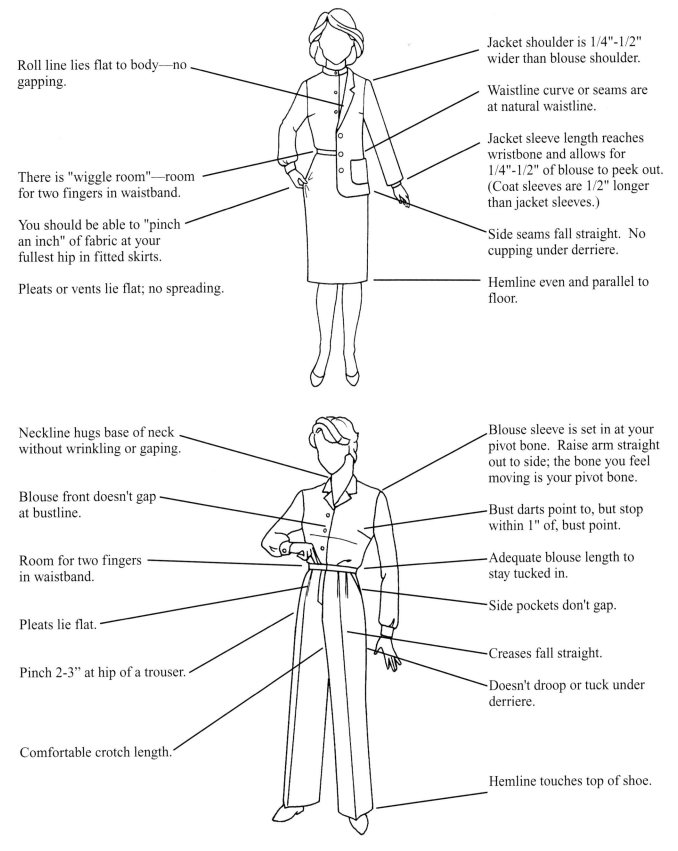

Roll line lies flat to body—no gapping.

Jacket shoulder is 1/4"-1/2" wider than blouse shoulder.

Waistline curve or seams are at natural waistline.

Jacket sleeve length reaches wristbone and allows for 1/4"-1/2" of blouse to peek out. (Coat sleeves are 1/2" longer than jacket sleeves.)

There is "wiggle room"—room for two fingers in waistband.

You should be able to "pinch an inch" of fabric at your fullest hip in fitted skirts.

Side seams fall straight. No cupping under derriere.

Pleats or vents lie flat; no spreading.

Hemline even and parallel to floor.

Neckline hugs base of neck without wrinkling or gaping.

Blouse sleeve is set in at your pivot bone. Raise arm straight out to side; the bone you feel moving is your pivot bone.

Blouse front doesn't gap at bustline.

Bust darts point to, but stop within 1" of, bust point.

Room for two fingers in waistband.

Adequate blouse length to stay tucked in.

Side pockets don't gap.

Pleats lie flat.

Pinch 2-3" at hip of a trouser.

Creases fall straight.

Doesn't droop or tuck under derriere.

Comfortable crotch length.

Hemline touches top of shoe.

Test the fit both standing and seated. Can you move freely in the garment?
Bend arms and lift them over your head.

Fabric Fundamentals

A few basic fabric facts can help you make sure that the great-looking garment in the store is an equally great performer in your wardrobe.

Fiber Facts

1. Fiber absorbency is a clue to comfort and durability.

   ♦ More-absorbent fibers are more comfortable to wear because they absorb body moisture and humidity. They are less prone to static electricity and will clean more easily.

   ♦ Less-absorbent fibers are less affected by body heat and moisture. They wrinkle less and hold their shape better. But they are less comfortable, more static prone and they pill more easily.

   Synthetic fibers like polyester, nylon, acetate and acrylic are less absorbent. Natural fibers like wool, linen, cotton and silk are more absorbent. Rayon, though a synthetic, is made from plant materials and is fairly absorbent.

2. The length of a fiber also affects appearance and performance.

   ♦ Long fibers are smooth and lustrous, wrinkle resistant, and pill resistant. Synthetics and natural silk are long fibers. The finest cotton and wool fibers are also long.

   ♦ Short fibers are soft and fuzzy, tend to pill, and wrinkle more easily. Most natural fibers are short, and some synthetics are cut into short lengths for a more natural appearance.

3. Manufacturers often blend fibers to decrease costs, increase prestige, increase washability, minimize wrinkling or add comfort and strength. It generally takes 35 percent of a fiber in a blend to make a significant difference, and 50 percent to get the most out of that fiber's good qualities. (A 5 percent Lycra blend, though, does add significant stretch.)

   ♦ A shirt of 65 percent cotton, 35 percent polyester will wrinkle less and wear better than an all-cotton shirt.

   ♦ A blend of opposite proportions (65 percent polyester, 35 percent cotton) will wrinkle even less and wear even longer, but will also be less comfortable to wear.

These fibers in a fabric...	Contribute...
Cotton or linen	Absorbency and comfort, minimum static buildup, better dye-ability
Wool	Bulk and warmth, absorbency, shape retention, wrinkle recovery
Silk	Luster, luxury, comfort
Mohair	Strength, luster, loopy texture
Cashmere/camel hair	Warmth, luxury, drapability, softness
Angora	Softness, fuzziness
Acrylic	Softness, wool-like qualities
Rayon	Absorbency, low static buildup, luster
Nylon	Strength, abrasion resistance, wrinkle resistance, lower cost
Acetate	Drapability, luster and shine, lower cost
Polyester	Wash-and-wear qualities, wrinkle resistance, shape retention, lower cost
Spandex	Elasticity and comfort

If you are unsure about care instructions, care as you would for the most sensitive fiber in the blend.

4. Fabric weave also affects durability and appearance.

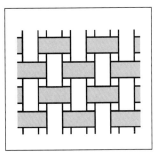

♦ Plain weave—Each yarn runs over one, under the next, producing a strong, firm fabric of any weight. Chiffon, gingham, flannel and challis are examples of this most common weave.

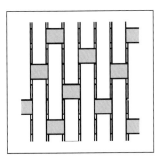

♦ Satin weave—Lengthwise yarns "float" over several crosswise ones to produce very lustrous fabric. These float yarns snag easily. Charmeuse and satin are examples of this fragile weave.

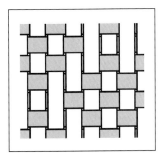

♦ Jacquard/dobby weaves—Figurative designs are produced by patterns of float threads. These are expensive to produce and can be fragile. Pique and brocade are examples.

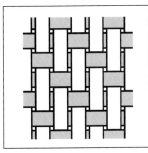

♦ Twill weave—A fine diagonal rib is formed in this weave. It is strong, resilient and wrinkle-resistant. Examples are denim and gabardine.

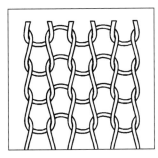

♦ Knits—The yarn is formed into a series of interlocking loops. Knits are durable, subject to only an occasional snag. And they are comfortable because of their stretchability.

How Can I Tell if This Fabric Will Work for Me?

1. Test wrinkle resistance and recover by crushing a corner of fabric in your hand and releasing it. Do the wrinkles stay or fall out quickly? The higher the natural fiber content, the more it will wrinkle. Woven fabrics wrinkle more than knits.

2. Check wearing qualities and shape retention. Stretch the fabric between thumbs and forefingers and hold for five seconds. If the yarns shift apart, strain on seams could be a problem. If the fabric doesn't spring back, the garment may stretch out of shape in wearing.

   Generally wovens hold their shape better than knits, and synthetics better than natural fibers.

3. Test the fabric for pilling. In an inconspicuous area of the garment, gently rub two layers of fabric right sides together. If this produces slight balls of fibers (called pills), the same thing will happen in abrasion areas when you wear the garment.

4. Check the fiber content for a comfort guide. In general, fabrics high in natural fibers are more comfortable. Synthetics often feel clammy because they don't breathe or absorb as well.

5. Check grain line. Lengthwise and crosswise threads should be at right angles to one another and lengthwise threads should run straight up and down the garment. Otherwise the garment will not hang evenly on your body.

   Invest in the best quality you can afford for your wardrobe basics. These coordinates need to be durable and make you look like a million.

Fabrics for Basic Skirts/Jackets/Pants

Fabric	Advantages	Disadvantages
Wool Gabardine	Wears extremely well. Comfortable because wool breathes and insulates. Lightweight gabs are seasonless, hold shape well, wrinkles hang out.	Expensive. Easily over-pressed. *Dry clean only.*
Wool Crepe	Drapes beautifully. Season-spanning comfort. Wrinkles hang out.	Expensive. Can snag. *Dry clean.*
Polyester Gabardine	Wrinkle-resistant, durable. Year-round wear except in hottest/coldest climates. Stays crisp, fresh. *Washable.*	Not quite as rich-looking as wool. Can snag or pill. Less comfortable than wool.
Linen and Silk Suitings	Generally wear well. Never pill. Absorbent and very comfortable. Dark colors are seasonless.	Lose body after repeated cleaning. Use spray sizing to restore body. Dark colors show wear more quickly. *Dry clean.*
Linen-like	Choose heavier weights for better wear. Blends of rayon, polyester, cotton and/or linen are less costly and more wrinkle-resistant than linen. *Washable.*	May pill. Loses body after washing or dry cleaning. Not as durable or rich-looking as pure linen.

Fabrics for Soft Skirts & Blouses

Fabric	Advantages	Disadvantages
Polyester Crepe de Chine	Drapes beautifully for fullness without bulk. Resists wrinkles. Very durable. *Machine wash.*	Nonabsorbent, can feel clammy. Subject to oily stains. Remove from dryer promptly to prevent heat-set wrinkles.
Silk Crepe de Chine	Superb drape and feel. Comfortable in all climates. Prints and dyes beautifully. *Hand wash or...*	Expensive. Subject to perspiration stains and damage. Wrinkles. *dry clean.*
Silk Broadcloth	Sportier, crisper and stronger than crepe de chine. Less expensive. *Hand washable.*	Susceptible to wrinkles and perspiration damage.
Silk Charmeuse	Shiny surface and soft drape. Dressy.	Can snag. *Dry clean.*
Cotton or Blended Broadcloth	More casual. Inexpensive. More comfortable than polyester. Wrinkles less than silk. *Washable.*	Higher cotton content, wrinkles more; higher polyester content, less comfortable.
Wool or Blend Challis	Lightweight and drapable. Usually a soft, warm brushed surface. *Most blends washable.*	Wool is more expensive, but durable. Polyester has tendency to pill.
Rayon Challis	Beautiful drape. Comfortable for year-round wear. *Usually washable.*	Retains new look longer if *dry cleaned.*

Additional Fabrics for Added Variety

Wool and Blended Flannel	Those with tight weave or hard finish wear best. Good winter basic in weights for all climates. *Blends usually less expensive and washable.*	Generally for winter only. Can be expensive. Less durable and more wrinkly than gabardine. Blends can pill or be scratchy. *Dry clean 100 percent wool.*
Wool Knit	Comfortable. Warm in winter. Lightweights drape beautifully. Heavier weights tailor well. *Sweaters may be hand washed.*	Expensive. Can snag. May stretch out of shape in wear, but can be pressed back. *Dry clean.*
Polyester Knits	Resist wrinkles; travel well. Hold their shape. Inexpensive. *Machine washable.*	Fiber doesn't breathe, so warm in summer; cold in winter. Subject to snags and oily stains.
Corduroy, Velvet, Velveteen	Very rich texture and color. *Some are washable.*	Not very durable; show wear and press marks easily. Can stretch out of shape, but will recover in washing or *dry cleaning.*
Ultrasuede Brand Fabrics	Elegant and very durable. Resist wrinkles. Hold shape well. Seasonless. *Machine washable.*	Very expensive. Warm in summer.

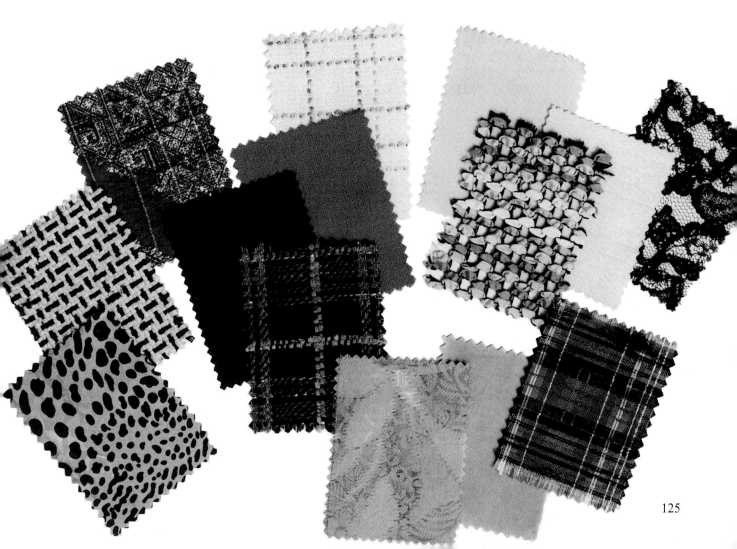

125

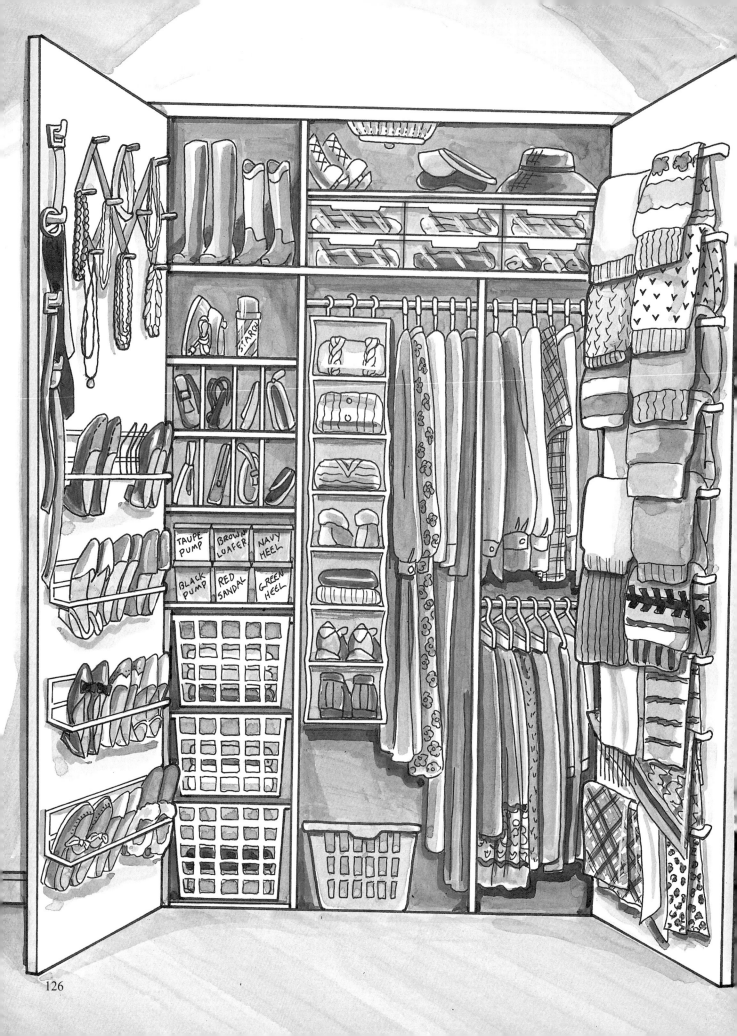

TAUPE
PUMP

BROWN
LOAFER

NAVY
HEEL

BLACK
PUMP

RED
SANDAL

GREEN
HEEL

STARCH

CHAPTER 10

Closet Control

To keep your wardrobe accessible, you should be able to see everything each time you open the closet door.

1. Hang everything you can. Don't put anything out of sight in a drawer if you can possibly hang it or stack it on open shelves.

2. Create two hanging levels so you can see bottoms in relation to tops. You'll be amazed how many new combinations suddenly appear.

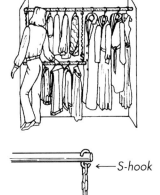

   Buy a system or make your own with screw eyes, S-hooks and chain.

← S-hook

← S-hook
← screw eye

3. Use the inside of doors for extra hanging space. Add a towel bar for sweaters or scarves, mug rack for jewelry, or a shoe rack.

4. See-through plastic boxes are great for dust-free shelf storage. Use the kind with slide-out drawers rather than lift-off lids.

5. Make your closet light and bright with a fresh coat of light-colored paint. If you lack lighting, you can bypass costly wiring and install a battery-operated light from the hardware store.

6. Keep your clothes organized by category and color. Review page 59 for specifics.

Safe Storage Strategies

Here are eight tips to minimize closet wear and tear on you wardrobe.

1. Don't crowd your closet. Let clothes hang freely to prevent wrinkling.

2. Fold stretchy bias garments and knit dresses over the hangers.

3. Take all your wire hangers back to the dry cleaners for recycling and replace them with some of these:

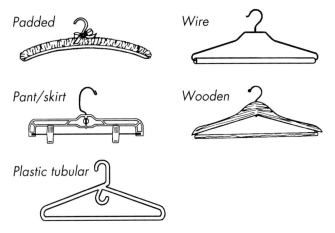

Padded   Wire

Pant/skirt   Wooden

Plastic tubular

4. Loops of tape sewn into the waistline of some dresses are intended to slip over the hanger hook and support the weight of the garment, preventing shoulder distortion. You can add them to other garments yourself.

5. Keep fragile items like lace, beads, velvet and suede in cloth bags for protection. Avoid plastic bags, which don't let the fabric breathe.

6. You can store sweaters right on hangers using this method introduced by image consultant Judith Rasband:

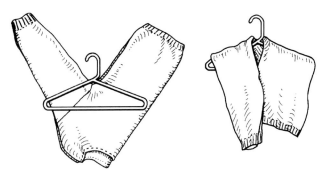

7. Avoid hanging fuzzy fabrics like mohair or fur next to ones that attract lint.

8. Clip-style skirt hangers can leave indentations in fine fabrics. Protect your garment by tucking a scrap of medium-weight fabric between the waistband and the clips.

Storage Solutions

Here are some specific ideas for hard-to-manage items:

1. Hang belts from:

- ♦ Cup hooks attached to the inside of the closet door or closet side wall

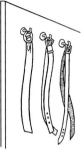

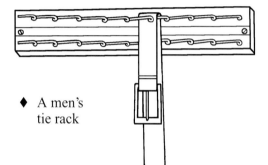

- ♦ A men's tie rack

2. Store scarves:

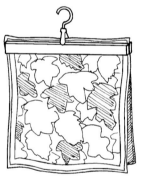

- ♦ Clipped to a skirt or pants hanger

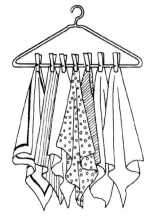

- ♦ Attach with clothes pins to a narrow metal hanger or towel bar

3. For jewelry:

- ♦ Mug rack

- ♦ Cutlery tray

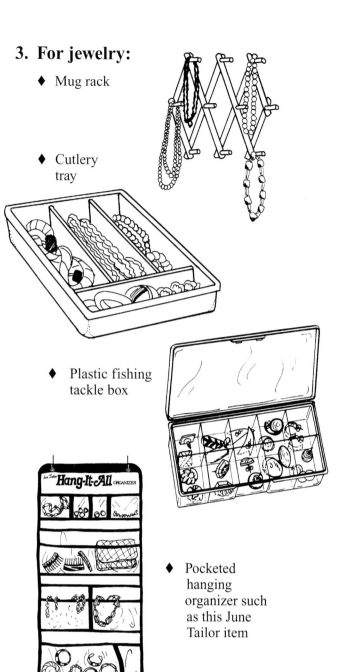

- ♦ Plastic fishing tackle box

- ♦ Pocketed hanging organizer such as this June Tailor item

4. Handle hosiery:

- ♦ In zip-top bags by color and style

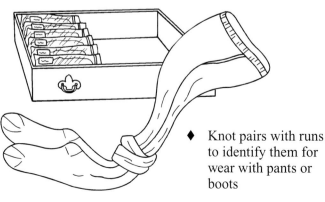

- ♦ Knot pairs with runs to identify them for wear with pants or boots

5. Handbags can go:

- ♦ Between vertical dividers on a shelf
- ♦ In free-standing wire baskets
- ♦ In a hanging purse and shoe caddy

6. Store shoes on:

- ♦ Free-standing or door-mounted rack
- ♦ Shelves in see-through plastic boxes
- ♦ Shelves in their own boxes, clearly labeled on the end with color and style
- ♦ Boot trees to prevent cracks when boots fold at the ankle

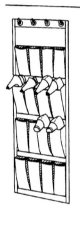

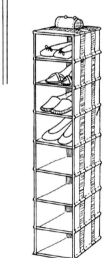

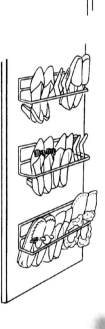

Out-of-Season Storage

- ♦ Store clothes in cool, dry areas to prevent mildew and out of direct sunlight to guard against fading.

- ♦ Create storage space by adding an extra high rod in a tall closet or a back rod in a deep closet.

- ♦ Garment racks and storage boxes can expand available space.

- ♦ Furs need professional reconditioning and cold storage off-season to prevent drying and cracking.

- ♦ Mothproofing is a MUST when temperatures exceed 50 degrees. Scatter moth balls liberally through stored items. Use layers of tissue paper to protect fabric from direct contact with mothballs. Keep storage area tightly sealed to hold in the vapors. NOTE: Don't use moth balls with leathers or furs.

- ♦ If you can't stand the moth ball smell, substitute cedar blocks or make one of these herbal blends instead. You'll find the ingredients at health food and/or craft stores. These mixes don't kill moth larvae, but they will repel egg-laying moths.

In your blender, make a powder of equal parts:

Sassafras	Thyme	Cloves
Lavender OR	Lavender OR	Caraway seeds
Dried rue	Woodruff	Nutmeg
Rosemary	Mace	Cinnamon
Toquin beans		

CHAPTER 11

Clothing Care

Quality clothes are worth protecting for longer life and better looks.

1. Air out clothes. Hang them outside the closet overnight so wrinkles fall out and odors dissipate. Dropping them in a pile results in more frequent cleaning, which causes unnecessary wear and expense.

2. Take a cue from men. Brush clothes to get rid of fiber-breaking dust...and dry clean only occasionally.

3. Let your clothes rest between wearings to regain their shape.

4. Mend small tears immediately, before they develop into bigger ones.

5. Remove pills with a "defuzzer" or whisk Dr. Scholl's® callous remover gently over the surface of the fabric.

6. Deodorant, perfume and lotions contain chemicals that damage fibers. Let them dry completely before you dress.

7. Stop runs with clear nail polish or Fray Check™. Prolong the life of nylons by painting the toe seam with Fray Check before wearing.

8. Apply clear nail polish to rough edges of jewelry to keep them from snagging clothes.

Removing Stains

1. Most spots can be removed completely with immediate action. The longer a spot sits, the harder it is to remove.

2. Never press over a spot; heat will set the stain.

3. Keep a spot remover on hand for quick saves on dry-clean garments.

4. Waiters and flight attendants swear by club soda to prevent stains from setting.

5. To remove a stain, put a clean cloth under the fabric, with the stain toward the cloth. Use soft fabric to dab stain remover or water through the stain until it is gone.

♦ Perspiration—on washables, pretreat by flushing with an ammonia/water solution. Rinse well.

♦ Ink—water-soluble hair spray dissolves ink on washables. Use rubbing alcohol on dry cleanables.

♦ Oils—on silks, pretreat and wash with Easy Wash®. On polyesters, pretreat with Spray 'N' Wash® and launder.

Wash or Dry Clean?

Read and follow the manufacturer's care label. Often a garment in a fabric you'd expect to be washable requires dry cleaning because of the interfacings or linings used inside.

Among washables, the finer the fabric, the more likely it should be hand washed and air dried rather than laundered by machine.

Handwashing Silk

1. To lukewarm water (100°) add a mild shampoo (silk is protein, like hair). Or use a cold water detergent like Wool Tone® by Van Wyck.

2. Swish garment for 1-2 minutes. Don't rub, twist or squeeze.

3. Rinse thoroughly in cold water (50°) to best remove soap and minimize wrinkling.

4. Lay wet garment on a towel and roll up to blot excess water.

5. Use a dry iron at a low setting to iron the garment dry.

Handwashing Wool Sweaters

1. To cool water, add a cold-water detergent like Wool Tone.

2. Very gently squeeze soapy water through sweater for 1-2 minutes, not 3. Rinse twice in cold water.

4. Pat out water, then roll in a towel and blot out excess moisture.

5. Dry sweater flat, blocking to original size if needed.

Machine Washing Delicates

1. Turn garments inside out to reduce abrasion on creases and edges.

2. Use the shortest wash cycle and lowest agitation speed available.

3. Use mesh laundry bags for pantyhose, lingerie and delicate blouses.

4. Over-drying can cause static, pilling, progressive shrinkage, wrinkling and puckered seams.

   ♦ Use warm, not hot, settings to warm fabric and remove wrinkles.

   ♦ Take clothes out of the dryer slightly damp and warm. Shake well and hang to cool and air dry.

   ♦ Tug gently on seams to stretch the thread and eliminate puckers.

Dry Cleaning— The Most for Your Money

1. Always clean both elements of a two-piece garment at the same time to avoid any color variation.

2. Point out spots and stains to your cleaner, and identify the cause. Also tell the cleaner the garment's fiber content.

3. Request ID tags attached with safety pins instead of staples.

4. Remove delicate buttons or cover them tightly with aluminum foil to prevent damage from cleaning chemicals.

5. Try bulk dry cleaning for items that don't require professional pressing. Priced by the pound, it can be a real money saver.

6. Over-pressing takes the life out of most fabrics and often leaves the imprint of seams and hems on the outside of the garment. Ask your cleaner for a soft or light press. Or request "dry clean only" and do your own touch-up pressing at home.

7. Plastic cleaner bags hold heat and attract moisture. Remove the bags before you put garments into the closet, so they can breathe.

8. Remember that most quality dry cleaners also offer clothing repair services, dyeing, water-repellancy treatment and other helpful services.

Pressing Matters

The right pressing equipment makes a big difference in the ease of the task and the finished appearance of the garment. You should have:

1. Good "shot-of-steam" iron with a nonstick coating and a visible water level indicator.

2. Well-padded ironing board. Use cotton canvas covers; metallic ones cause heat to bounce back and can damage delicate fabrics.

3. Sleeve board* and pressing mitt* make it easy to press sleeves without creases. They also help reach hard-to-press areas.

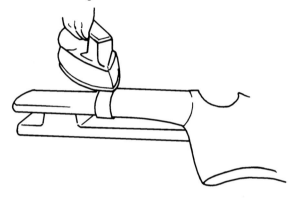

4. Seam roll* allows you to prevent unsightly ridges when you press seams open after laundering or cleaning. Because the seam roll is curved and the bottom of the iron is flat, the garment curves away from the iron so you press only the seam and not the edge of the seam allowance.

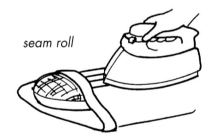

seam roll

5. Cotton see-through press cloth* prevents fabric shine, but lets you see what you're doing.

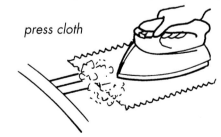

press cloth

*Available in fabric stores.

6. Hot iron cleaner keeps your soleplate clean and smooth. Use it on a hot iron with several layers of damp cloth, as directed.

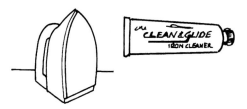

7. Soleplate cover makes it easy to press synthetics without creating shine. Remove it from your iron periodically to clear away lint buildup and to clean the soleplate.

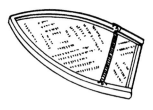

Pressing Pointers

1. Always test iron temperature in a hidden area of the garment first. A too-hot iron can literally melt holes in synthetic fabrics.

2. Press delicate fabrics on the wrong side or use a press cloth or soleplate cover for top pressing.

3. Use a little spray starch or sizing to keep cotton, linen or lace looking crisp.

4. Fabrics have memory only when cool. Allow garments to cool before you move them, or the creases you just pressed will fall out.

5. Eliminate daily touch-up pressing by choosing tomorrow's outfit tonight and letting it hang outside the closet. Any closet wrinkles will fall out overnight.

The Bottom Line

Shoes and boots can last for years with proper care, and the same is true for handbags and briefcases.

1. Give leather shoes a paste polish before the first wearing and future stains will penetrate less easily.

2. Waterproof shoes with a silicone protector available at shoe stores and repair shops.

3. Clean patent leather and vinyl with a soft cloth dampened in white vinegar. Dry and shine with a soft cloth.

4. Protect suede with a stain repellent spray. Use an art-gum eraser or special suede cleaning bar to remove minor soil. Rub stubborn stains with very fine sandpaper. Restore the surface with a suede brush.

5. If shoes or boots get wet, stuff them with tissue or newsprint and let them dry slowly away from direct heat. Polish when dry.

6. Prevent salt damage by wiping immediately with a 50/50 solution of white vinegar and water. Repair shops also sell a commercial salt remover.

7. Shoes last longer if you let them rest between wearings to air out perspiration and moisture that can harden the inner shoe. Stuff with tissue, toe shapes or shoe trees to maintain shape.

8. Replace heel tips as soon as wear begins to show. Consider resoling fine shoes if the uppers are in good shape. It's far cheaper than buying new. You can also have scuffed uppers re-dyed to a darker color.

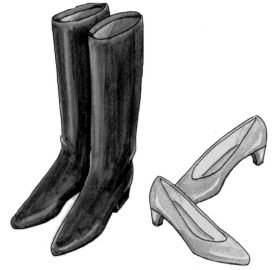

CHAPTER 12
So You Sew

Sewing enthusiasts have some special advantages when it comes to building effective wardrobes.

♦ When you need an exact color or specific figure-flattering style.

♦ When you need a specialized fit for your unique shape.

♦ When you need an item that isn't currently in season.

Whatever the need...YOU CAN SEW IT!!

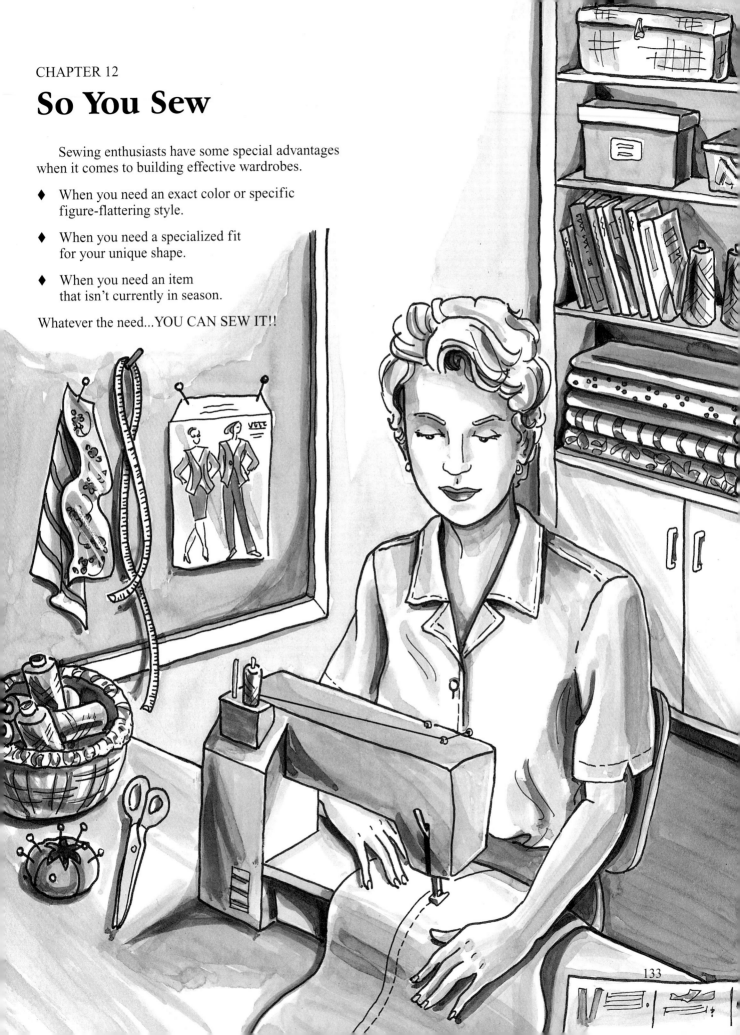

I've noticed some typical wardrobing weaknesses many of us seem to share. Do any of these describe you?

1. **Overlooking ourselves**. We can get so excited about a particularly interesting fabric combination or intricate pattern detail that we leap right into a project without ever considering how the finished garment will suit US.

   If that sounds familiar, review the Getting To Know You section to develop the habit of putting yourself into the planning picture.

2. **Getting "over-printy"**. Let's face it...prints, plaids and textured fabrics are much more enticing on the bolt than a plain solid. But those solids make up the workhorse items in any wardrobe.

   Too many prints equals too few wardrobe combinations. Discipline yourself to sew more solids for a more versatile wardrobe.

3. **Doting on details**. An intricately styled jacket with detailed seaming, contrasting piping, buttons and trims may showcase our sewing abilities. But it probably won't mix as well in our wardrobes as a more streamlined style.

   As a rule, simple styles sewn in fabulous fabrics will give you the best return on your sewing time investment.

4. **Under-accessorizing**. Since we spend more shopping time in fabric stores than in department stores, we often miss the message that accessories are necessary to complete any fashion look. Review Chapter 6 (page 85) carefully to absorb this important wardrobe lesson.

5. **Becoming TOO thrifty**. There's nothing wrong with appreciating the savings sewing offers. But fight the tendency to become downright CHEAP. Treat yourself to the very finest fabrics you can afford. They will cooperate with you in the construction process. And they'll last for years in your wardrobe too.

6. **Believing you have to sew EVERYTHING** in your wardrobe. Even industry professionals recognize that today's busy lifestyles make it impossible to sew everything you wear.

To Sew or Buy?

It Makes Sense To Sew...

1. When you can't find what you want in ready-to-wear. Choosing your own combination of fabric and pattern vastly increases your options.

2. When you can make the item in less time than it would take you to shop for it.

3. When you're capable of creating better quality clothing than you could afford ready-made.

4. When your body proportions make it difficult to find a good fit in a ready-made garment.

5. When you find expensive items that would be easy to copy.

6. When you can create a big impact by sewing simple styles in smashing fabrics.

It Makes Sense To Buy...

1. When your time is worth more than the money saved by making the garment.

2. When you don't have time to make what you need.

3. When the details or the fabric are beyond your skills.

4. When the color, fit and styling are great for you...and so is the price.

5. When you find a great item at a great price—even if it needs minor adjustments in fit or detail. With basic sewing skills, you can easily upgrade a bargain by...

   ◆ Replacing average buttons with distinctive ones
   ◆ Adding a fashionable belt
   ◆ Redoing poorly stitched hems
   ◆ Changing the length for a better proportion
   ◆ Adding or replacing trims
   ◆ Adding or removing shoulder pads for smoother fit
   ◆ Tapering side seams for closer-to-the-body fit

A Third Option— Hire a Professional Dressmaker

Have clothing made to beautifully fit your body and your personal style. See the Resource List, page 155, for information about the Professional Association of Custom Clothiers.

Organize Your Fabric Stash

Many sewing enthusiasts have discovered that, even when they can't find time to sew...there's always time to buy more fabric! But before your next shopping expedition, beg, borrow or steal some time to organize your current fabric stash.

Clean House

Do a clean-out of your fabric stash, just like you did with the clothes in your closet.

♦ Check color first. If it's not in your palette, discard it. Or try dyeing it to a more flattering shade.

♦ Tastes change. If you no longer love it, get rid of it.

♦ Evaluate prints carefully. They are easily outdated; discard anything that isn't current.

♦ Consider the weight of the fabric. Bulky or heavily textured fabrics add visual pounds... so discard anything that isn't flattering.

Dispose of Your Discards Immediately

♦ Have a swap meet. Invite sewing friends to trade or buy.

♦ Include the discards in a garage sale.

♦ Charities are grateful recipients of fabrics, and it's worth a tax deduction for you.

Catalog What's Left

Here's one easy system:

1. Glue a swatch of each piece to its own 3x5 card.

2. Record additional information as shown at right.

3. Store all cards in a zip-top bag, organized in any order that makes sense for you:

by color   by fiber content
by fabric type   by weight
by season   (top/bottom)
by end use

Now Use Your System

♦ Use your file as a guide for planning new projects so they will blend with what you have.

♦ Take the file with you any time you shop or travel.

♦ Select your next sewing project by comparing your file pages with your current wardrobe and finding possible coordinates.

Store Your Stash Efficiently

1. Preshrink fabrics before you put them away. Snip one corner on the diagonal to label the piece preshrunk.

2. Designate a fabric closet. Remove the bar, add floor-to-ceiling shelves, then store fabrics by color, weight or end use.

3. Very crisp or deep pile fabrics are better rolled than folded to avoid creases. Ask your fabric store for empty cardboard tubes.

4. Organize your interfacings:

♦ Discard any old unidentifiable fusible interfacings.

♦ Stock up on your favorites in 5-10 yard lengths. They will cut to better advantage, and you'll always have a selection on hand.

♦ Roll fusible interfacings and their plastic instruction sheets onto cardboard tubes to avoid creasing.

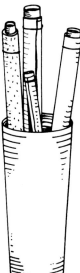

Fabric name _____ attach swatch here

Fiber content _____

Width ____ Yardage ____

Care Instructions _____

Storage Location _____

5. What about scraps?

♦ Toss anything that isn't big enough to make something...at least a scarf or bow.

♦ Roll the "keepers" in large boxes, sorted by color or fabric type.

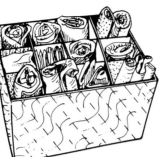

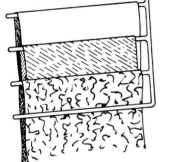

June Tailor 3-Way Thread Rack

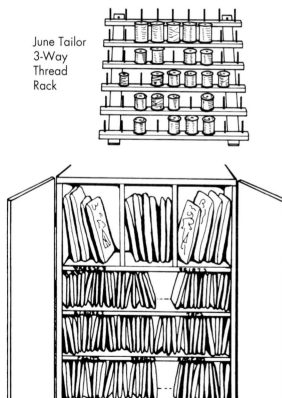

*For additional organization ideas see the Palmer/Pletsch book **Dream Sewing Spaces** (page 158).*

6. Store patterns efficiently:

♦ Back favorite patterns with fusible interfacing for durability. Keep the pieces and the original envelope in a large zip-top bag.

♦ Or store pattern pieces in a manila file folder and glue the original envelope to the face of the folder.

♦ Store patterns by style in a file cabinet or cardboard file box.

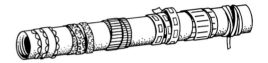

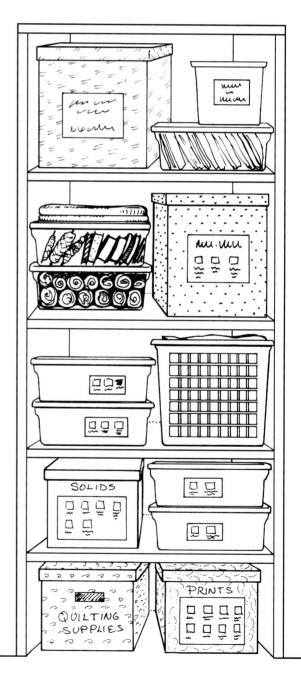

Shopping for Fabric Capsules

Plan ahead for wardrobe versatility by selecting your fabric in groupings, with a capsule of coordinating garments in mind. This capsule concept is far easier to execute in a fabric store than in a clothing boutique where you might find the right colors and fabrics, but made into the wrong styles.

1. Select a top-quality bottom-weight fabric in a favorite solid color for matching jacket, skirt and pants.

2. Carry that bolt around the store to find coordinating top weights for blouses and two-piece dresses. No coordinates? Pick a new solid and start again.

3. When you have a whole group of coordinating possibilities, check to see if any of the prints introduce new colors that you could repeat in additional solid fabrics. Add those new solids, if you can find them, to your group.

   Spread out all the "possibles" and mix and match them until you narrow the selection to the pieces you need.

   Don't forget to compare them with your swatches of current clothes and fabric on hand. You'll probably find even more combinations there.

5. Buy it all at once, to avoid disappointment later and guard against seasonal color changes. Of course you don't have to sew it all this week. But remember that selecting simple pattern styles will showcase those beautiful fabrics and speed your construction time as well.

6. If you haven't selected specific patterns for each item, use these guidelines for amounts to buy:

	45" Fabric	54-60" Fabric
Slim skirt	2x finished length plus 8" for hem, waistband	finished length plus 6"
Dirndl skirt	same	same
Pants	same	same
Long-sleeve blouse	2 1/4 yards	1 1/2 yards
Shell blouse	1 yard	1 yard
Hip-length jacket	3 yards	2 yards

Smart Shopping In Pattern Catalogs

1. Scan all major brands to see trends. Note patterns you like by style number and page number. If you see similar styles in several catalogs, compare prices.

2. Carefully study the front editorial pages for the season's newest trends in styles, colors, wardrobe coordination and accessories.

3. There are hundreds of designs in each catalog, but they are grouped by category, and the newest designs are photographed in the introductory pages and are placed near the front of their respective categories.

4. To make room for new styles added each month, slow sellers are discontinued quarterly. A pattern shown in a half-page illustration may be on its way out. If you like it, buy it now.

5. Patterns labeled "easy" contain fewer pieces and simplified instructions. But any pattern can be fast if it has these details:

   ◆ Gathers instead of darts or pleats

   ◆ Few details like plackets, yokes, topstitching

   ◆ Neckline finishes like binding or facing instead of a collar

   ◆ No pieces cut on the bias

6. The small line drawings show to-scale proportions, design details and seamlines. Consider carefully how those lines will look on YOUR body. What areas will the lines emphasize?

7. Suggested fabrics are those most suitable for the design.

   ◆ A pattern labeled "knits only" requires a stretchable fabric to give the ease necessary for comfortable fit.

   ◆ A pattern labeled "Not suitable for plaids" includes pattern shapes that prevent the plaid lines from matching at major seams.

The Pattern Envelope

1. The envelope front shows you the various views. Fashion sketches drawn on idealized model figures don't provide much insight into true garment proportions. But they do offer wardrobe coordinating possibilities and accessory ideas.

2. Line drawings of the back views show the true proportions and design details.

3. Finished garment lengths and widths are listed in the yardage chart or the instruction sheet inside. They help you know how much fullness to expect. Compare these measurements to garments you already know are flattering. If the fullness allowed is more than you prefer, consider choosing the next smaller pattern size.

4. Garment descriptions give you information about fit and details that may not be obvious from the pictures, such as "dropped shoulders" or "blouson."

Patterns are made to body measurements plus standard wearing ease (wiggle room). Most patterns also include additional design ease to create the fashion look. The following terms are used to indicate the amount of ease allowed in a pattern, and the fashion drawings are examples of those descriptive terms.

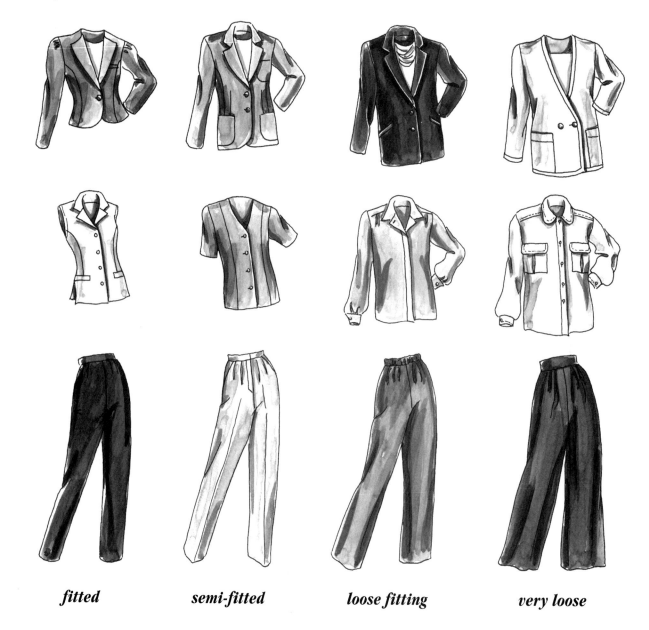

fitted   *semi-fitted*   *loose fitting*   *very loose*

Creative Combinations

Successfully combining pattern and fabric is the most creative part of sewing. It can also be the most challenging. You can use either the pattern or the fabric as your starting point.

Starting With the Pattern

When you have an itemized list of wardrobe needs, select patterns first. You can look for specific styling and details, then find the right fabric. You have more freedom in style choice when you aren't limited by the characteristics of a fabric you've already purchased.

The following steps will help you find the right fabric for your pattern:

1. Check the list of suggested fabrics on the pattern envelope. The sketches or photos of the style are additional clues.

    ♦ Is it shown in a solid or print?

    ♦ Does the style need a soft fabric to fall gracefully or a crisp one to hold a defined shape?

    ♦ Look at similar styles in boutiques or catalogs for additional fabric clues.

2. If some of the suggested fabrics aren't available, substitute the same way you might in a recipe. Look for other fabrics with similar weight and drape as those listed.

3. Preview the finished garment by draping the fabric on your body to simulate the design.

    ♦ If the design has gathers, gather the fabric with your hands.

    ♦ Do the gathers fall softly or stand away from your body?

    ♦ Would the fabric drape better on the bias?

"Try on" the fabric before you buy to check color, drape, experiment with style ideas.

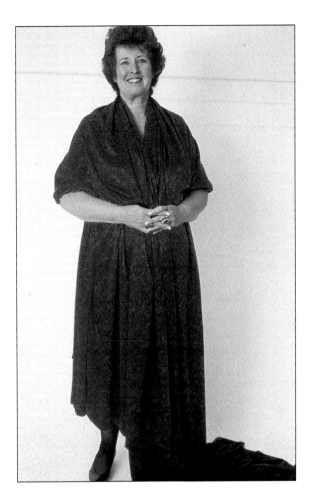

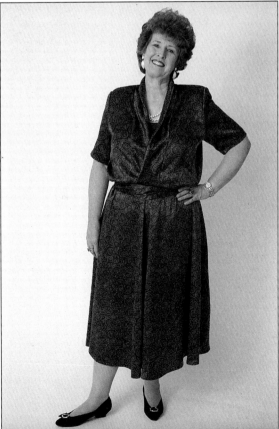

Starting With Fabric

1. If you're selecting a pattern for a print or plaid, be sure there are no restrictions for these fabrics on the back of the envelope.

   ♦ Almost any style will work with a small all-over print, but large prints usually require simple styles. Design details would just get lost in the large print.

   ♦ One-way designs and prints with obvious motifs look best when they can be matched at major seamlines.

3. Crisp fabrics lend themselves to tailored styles with darts and seams to shape them to body contours.

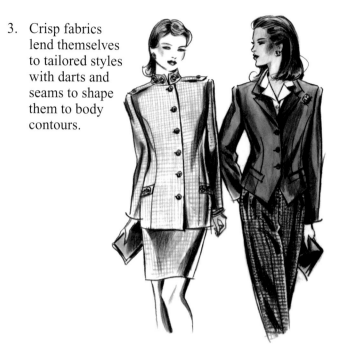

4. Soft, fluid, lightweight fabrics work best in designs with few details and more fullness and drape.

5. The softer and more drapable the fabric, the more fullness you can use without getting a bulky look. A gathered skirt that would work beautifully in challis would be bulky in corduroy.

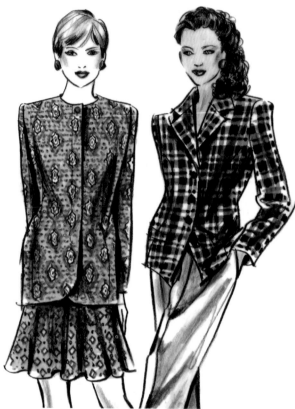

2. Solid fabrics can take more pattern seaming and details. Construction details show to best advantage in flannel, gabardine, jersey, silk and linen.

140

6. Sheer fabrics require simple designs, few seams and limited details.

7. Pile fabrics like velvet and corduroy are easiest to sew in styles with minimum detailing.

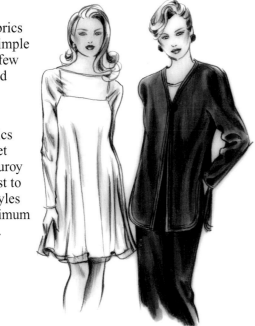

8. Border prints and embroideries limit pattern choices, but with creativity, the results can be exciting.

   ♦ Seam blouse at center front, creating a double border. Repeat on the center seam of the skirt.

   ♦ Asymmetrical vertical placement of a border is a flattering, lengthening effect.

   ♦ Place an eyelet edge at hem, sleeve edge and collar.

   ♦ Use a border to jazz up a simple vest.

   ♦ Use a border across the shoulder area to create the effect of a yoke.

Check Your Choices

If you can answer "Yes" to most of these questions, you have planned a wardrobe winner. If not, perhaps your plan needs modifications.

☐ Does this project fill a need in my wardrobe? Impulse purchases usually aren't a wise use of your dollar.

☐ Is the color one of my personal best?

☐ Will this item work with at least three things in my present wardrobe?

☐ Do I own the necessary accessories to complete the look? If not, am I willing to buy them?

☐ If I've worn this fiber before, was it comfortable?

☐ Am I willing to care for this fabric as the manufacturer recommends?

☐ Are the print and/or texture of the fabric flattering to me?

☐ Do the lines of the pattern enhance my figure assets and minimize my challenge areas?

☐ Are the construction details within my sewing abilities?

☐ If I have worn a similar style before, was it comfortable and flattering?

☐ Is it on the upswing of the fashion curve so I can wear it long enough to get full value for the time and money I plan to spend?

☐ Does the total cost plus the sewing time required fit my time/money budget?

Be Your Own Designer

You can get great mileage by using a favorite pattern again and again. And no one will suspect, if you individualize each garment with new fashion details.

There are many good reasons to reuse patterns.

♦ Patterns today are costly.

♦ You made all the necessary alterations the first time.

♦ You are familiar with the construction steps.

♦ You know for sure the style looks good on you.

Sewing is easier the second time around if you record the following:

♦ Date sewn

♦ Weight and body measurements

♦ Adjustments made to pattern

♦ Fabric and interfacing used

Vary the look of a repeat-performance pattern by choosing fabrics with an entirely different mood.

2. Velvet skirt and cardigan, beaded lace shell

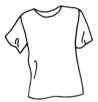

basic shell

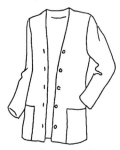

cardigan jacket

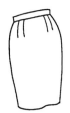

slim skirt

1. Summer print skirt and shell, linen jacket

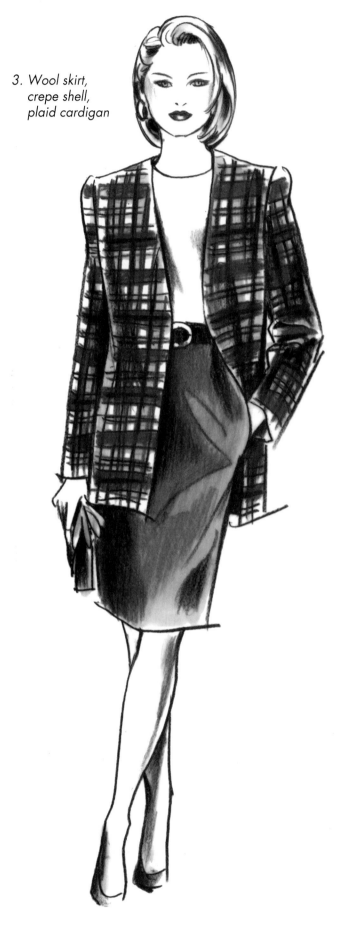

*3. Wool skirt,
   crepe shell,
   plaid cardigan*

Individualize a basic blazer with one of these ideas:

♦ Round the lapels and collar ends. Use a French curve for consistent shaping.

♦ Eliminate back and sleeve vents for a dressier look.

♦ Add elbow patches and sew the pocket flaps and upper collar from matching Ultrasuede brand fabric.

♦ Topstitch narrow ribbon or braid onto the collar and sleeve edges before sewing the seams.

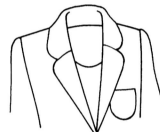

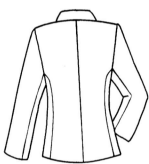

French curve

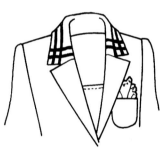

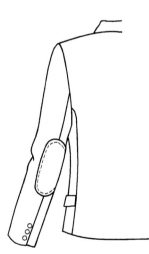

Customize a Blouse Pattern

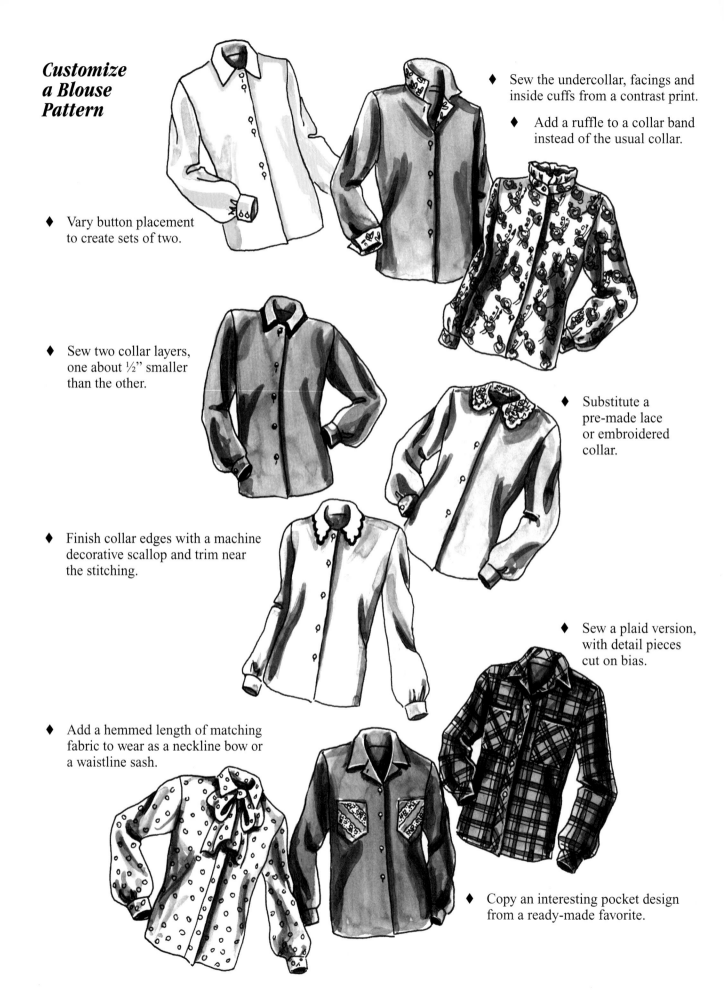

♦ Vary button placement to create sets of two.

♦ Sew two collar layers, one about ½" smaller than the other.

♦ Finish collar edges with a machine decorative scallop and trim near the stitching.

♦ Add a hemmed length of matching fabric to wear as a neckline bow or a waistline sash.

♦ Sew the undercollar, facings and inside cuffs from a contrast print.

♦ Add a ruffle to a collar band instead of the usual collar.

♦ Substitute a pre-made lace or embroidered collar.

♦ Sew a plaid version, with detail pieces cut on bias.

♦ Copy an interesting pocket design from a ready-made favorite.

Fashion Make-Over How-Tos

In Chapter 4, The Wardrobe Workout, we introduced the idea of fashion make-overs of the garments in your closet (pages 58-59). Even a novice sewer can handle minor updates on current garments. Start by collecting this basic equipment:

The Basic Necessities

♦ Sharp 8" dressmaker shears

♦ Sharp embroidery scissors

♦ Hand needles, size 10 sharps for hems

♦ Round head pins

♦ Seam ripper

♦ Measuring tools—tape measure, yardstick, sewing gauge

♦ Flat skirt hooks in black and silver

And you certainly will enjoy these handy extras:

♦ Grabbit®—a magnetic pin catcher with a wide, shallow surface to hold lots of pins. Turn it over to pick up spilled pins too.

♦ Fray Check™—liquid ravel preventer. Run a thin coating along a fabric edge for a permanent seam finish. Stop runs in nylons too.

♦ Glue stick— "baste" buttons and trims in place for easy sewing. Washes out.

♦ Pinch-and-pull bodkin—great for replacing elastic

♦ Seams Great®/Seam Saver®—pre-cut strips of nylon tricot. Pull on the strip and it folds over the edge of a fabric. Zigzag in place for a neat seam finish.

♦ Basting tape—narrow double-stick tape that replaces hand basting. Great for zippers, matching plaids.

♦ Erasable fabric markers in light or dark color. Some erase with a damp cloth, others disappear on their own in 24-48 hours.

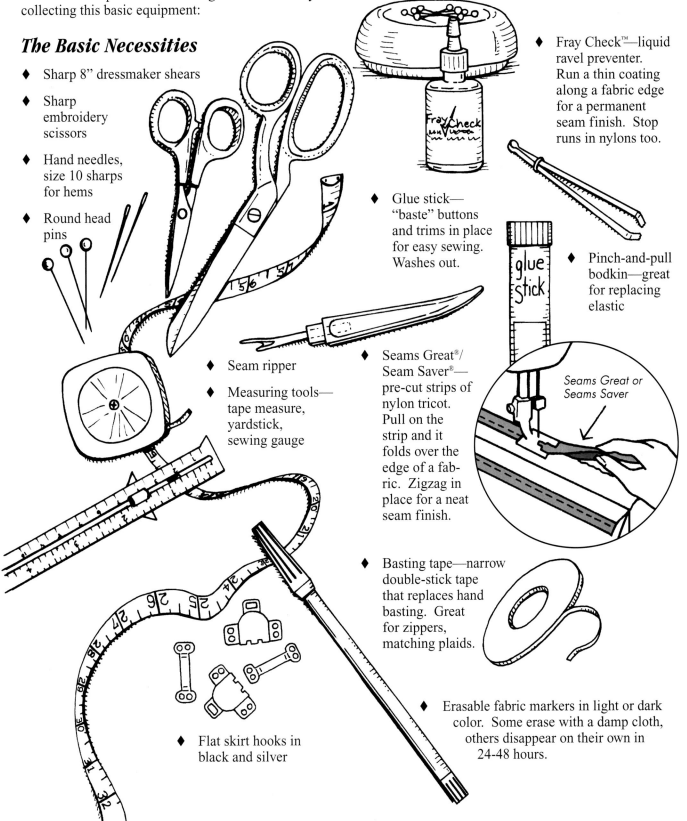

Seams Great or Seams Saver

Perfect Hems

The right hem or sleeve length can make the difference between dowdy and dynamite. Changes of even 1/4" can have a big impact.

To Create the Perfect Hem:

1. Carefully remove the old stitches with a seam ripper or small scissors.

2. Try on the garment and mark the desired new length, measuring up from the floor evenly all around.

3. Press in the new hem edge lightly.

4. Cut off excess fabric length. Hem depth should be between 1 1/2" and 2" in most garments.

5. Trim seams within the hem allowance to 1/4".

6. Finish the hem edge with one of the following:

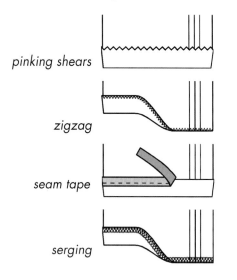

pinking shears

zigzag

seam tape

serging

7. Use the hand blind stitch, which never leaves a ridge on the outside.

   ♦ Size 10 sharp needles let you catch only a fiber of the outside fabric so hemming stitches won't show.

   ♦ A single strand of polyester thread provides the strongest, longest-lasting stitches.

   ♦ Fold down 1/4" of the hem edge and stitch between the two layers. Use a loose running stitch at least 1/2" long, catching only a fiber of the outside fabric.

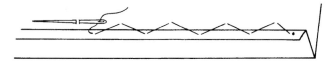

Other Ways to Shorten

Use Tucks

They are ideal for straight or dirndl skirts in lightweight fabrics. And they are far easier than shortening a sleeve from the cuff or the armhole. Two or more tucks create a more balanced look.

1. Mark tuck stitching lines with a water-erasable marker. Use a sewing gauge to maintain even spacing.

2. Pin or baste in place.

3. Try on to double-check the revised length.

4. Stitch permanently and press.

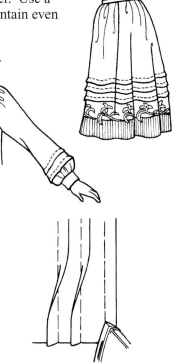

Shorten from the Top

This is ideal for border prints because it doesn't disturb the bottom edge. It works well when you want a little more waistline room too.

1. Remove the waistband and zipper.

2. Cut away excess length from the top edge, leaving a 5/8" seam allowance.

3. Lengthen darts or change them to soft gathers.

4. Replace the zipper and waistband.

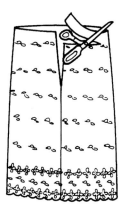

Lengthening

1. Remove the old hem and press out the crease.

2. For stubborn creases, try a mixture of half water and half white vinegar on a press cloth. The vinegar helps unset the old crease.

3. Mark the desired new length and press.

4. Stitch the hem as described on the previous page.

5. If the crease still shows, add several parallel rows of topstitching to camouflage it.

For Too-Short Pants

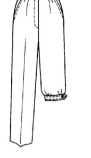

♦ Cut off 2" below the knee and make knickers, using the trimmed-away fabric to make the bottom bands.

♦ Cut off at the hemline and add purchased ribbing for cuffs.

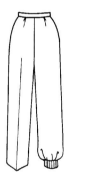

♦ Shorten fuller pants into Bermudas or city shorts.

Transforming Culottes

Turn full pants or culottes into a skirt. Remove the inseam stitches and sew new front and back seams straight down from just above the crotch curve. Trim the seam allowance to 5/8" and press open. Hem.

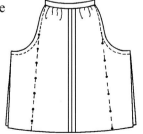

Tapering

A-line or straight skirts and fuller pants can be much more flattering if they taper at the hemline.

1. Unstitch the hem.

2. Pin or baste new side seams, starting just below the full hip and tapering toward the hemline.

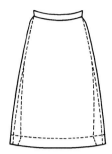

3. For pants, pin along both the inseam and outseam.

4. Try on to test the new width.

5. Stitch the new seams, tapering back outward in the hem allowance.

6. Restitch the hem and press.

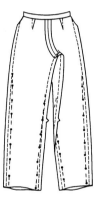

Instant Taper

Hand-stitch an inverted pleat at the bottom of a pant leg for a dressy, skinny look.

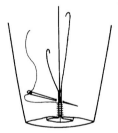

Make More Room

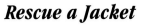
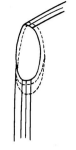

When an armhole is too snug, stitch the underarm seam 1/4" deeper. Trim the seam to 1/4". Try on the garment and repeat the alteration if still more room is required.

Pants that are too snug in the crotch can be altered the same way. Stitch the crotch curve 1/4" lower, trim and try on. Repeat if still more room is needed.

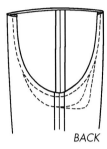

BACK

For more room in the seat only, stitch the center back seam lower.

Shoulder Secrets

♦ Add shoulder pads if you have these wrinkles:

♦ Remove or reduce shoulder pads if you have these:

♦ Try on the garment and adjust pad to the proper position. Pin the pad in place from the outside, extending it 1/4-1/2" into the sleeve cap. On the inside, loosely hand-tack the pad to the shoulder seam allowance and armhole seam allowances.

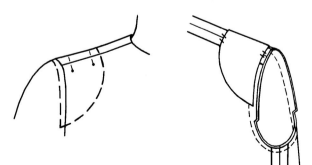

♦ Use the foam shoulder pads that rest directly on your shoulder and are held in place by the weight of the garment.

Rescue a Jacket

Cover worn jacket elbows with pre-cut leather patches...or cut your own from Ultrasuede fabric.

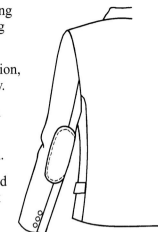

♦ Unstitch the sleeve lining hem and push the lining up out of the way.

♦ Pin the patch into position, centered over the elbow.

♦ Hand or machine stitch the patch in place.

♦ Restitch the lining hem.

♦ Add Ultrasuede-covered buttons to pull the look together.

If a jacket style is too boxy to flatter your body shape, taper the side seams at the waist. Pin the alteration and try it on before stitching.

For even more shaping, add lengthwise darts front and back. For other jacket ideas see pages 41 and 143.

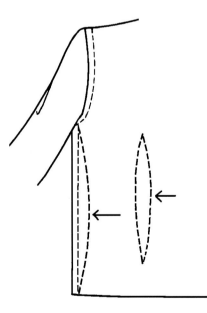

Shirt Savers

For frayed or outdated shirt collars:

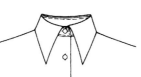

- Remove the stitching at the top of the band.

- Pull out the collar and discard it.

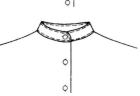

- Restitch the top edge of the band.

For variety, insert a narrow lace or eyelet between the band layers before restitching.

Or use the old collar as a pattern to cut a new one from contrasting fabric. Insert the new collar between the band layers and restitch. Make matching new cuffs to tie in the new color.

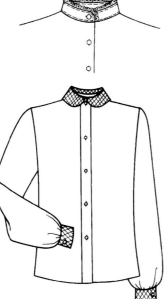

If the lower edge of the cuff is frayed:

- Turn under 1/4" to the wrong side and topstitch.

- Add a narrow ribbon or braid trim.

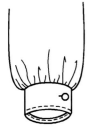

- Cut off the sleeve just above the placket. Hem the lower edge and roll up the sleeve.

Tricks With Trims

Use lace, appliques, ribbon, Ultrasuede scraps or decorative trim to camouflage stains, cigarette burns or moth holes.

Insert lace strips on a silky blouse. "Baste" with a glue stick, then hand or machine stitch. Cut away fabric underneath if desired.

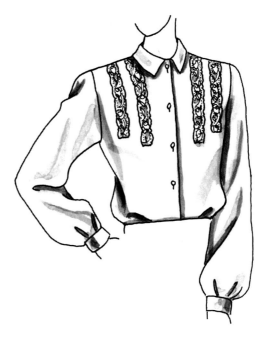

Stitch on appliques to cover stains. Repeat on cuffs for design unity.

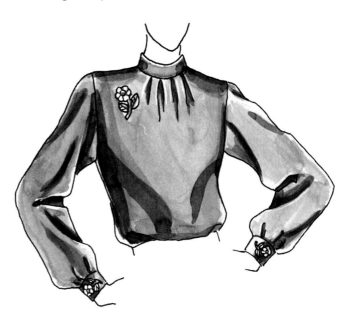

Lacy hankie points can be appliqued to a blouse front, collar or cuffs by hand or machine.

A pretty floral trim can hide moth holes or stains on a sweater.

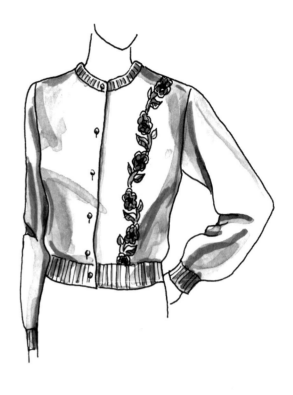

Cover a stained neckline or cuff edge with bias binding.

Cover worn edges of a jacket collar/lapel with braid or binding. Repeat on sleeve edge.

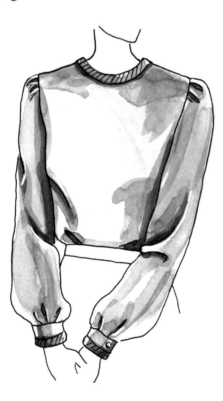

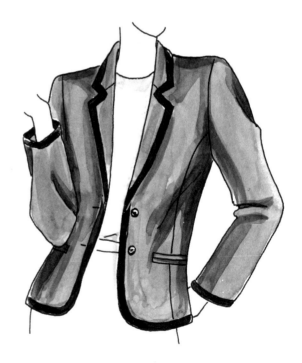

CHAPTER 13
Looking Good On The Go

Cartoon images of a foolish female traveling with 17 suitcases are hopelessly out of date. "Lean and mean" is the name of the game for today's traveler.

One suit and several blouses can get a professional woman through a week of business travel. And the same concept works equally well for pleasure trips.

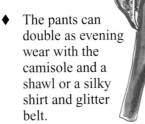

♦ Start with a basic skirt and jacket. Add matching pants or an alternate skirt.

♦ The pants can double as evening wear with the camisole and a shawl or a silky shirt and glitter belt.

♦ The cardigan can go casual with the pants, or create a softer suit look with a solid skirt.

♦ Pack a two-piece print dress. It will provide a blouse with the suit as well as a jacketed dress look. With dressier accessories, it can go right into evening. Choose a quality polyester fabric, jersey or interlock knit, ideally one that you can hand wash in the hotel sink.

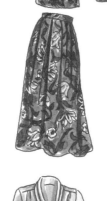

♦ Add an assortment of tops including a silky blouse, basic cardigan sweater and a camisole.

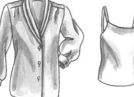

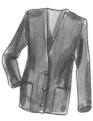

It Pays to Plan

1. Make a list of anticipated activities and what you'll need to wear for each.

2. Consolidate whenever possible. Even if you see the same people, they'll admire your know-how.

3. If you buy a new wardrobe for a big trip, wear everything at least once before you go, to work out any snags and identify needed accessories.

Plan Major Pieces First

♦ Use neutral colors for your main pieces so everything goes with everything. Darker neutrals and prints camouflage minor soil and wrinkles.

♦ Pack easy-care fabrics like washable, drip-dry synthetics.

Knits earn an A+ for packability. Wool flannels, tweeds and gabardines pack well. And Ultrasuede brand fabric is lightweight and wrinkle-free.

♦ Every top should go with every bottom. Extra tops are lightweight to pack, and extend your wardrobe options.

♦ Include a lightweight dark pant that can go from day to evening. Black is the universal pant color for evening and can be teamed with tops in any color. If your coloring is warm, substitute a rich dark brown or teal.

♦ Pack items that can do double duty, like a blouse that can double as a shirt-jacket.

♦ Expect weather extremes and plan clothing layers you can add or subtract accordingly.

♦ Choose your coat for the climate of your destination, but always be prepared for rain. A nylon cire raincoat can roll into a tiny corner of your tote bag. Water-resistant Ultrasuede is a perfect all-weather choice too.

A Security Tip

To protect yourself from pickpockets or theives, wear a shoulder bag with the strap *over* your head and across your body. Be sure the strap is the correct length for the bag to hang at the top of your hip bone...and in *front* of your body, where you can watch it. As an alternative, wear a hip pack, again with the storage area at the front of your body.

The Necessary Extras

♦ Accessories change the look of basic pieces. Use color accents in scarves, belts and jewelry to spice up your neutrals.

♦ Don't risk losing your valuable fine jewelry. Take only what you will wear and wear it all the time.

♦ Shoes are heavy, so limit yourself to a comfortable day shoe and one evening pair. Substitute comfy socks for bedroom slippers.

♦ Take one handbag that works with everything and pack a flat clutch for evening. Consider a lightweight fold-away tote bag for sightseeing and souvenir shopping.

♦ Airplanes can be chilly, so tuck a sweater and socks into your carry-on bag.

♦ Get triple mileage from a cotton knit jumpsuit. It's casualwear for around the hotel, a swim cover-up and even sleepwear...all in one garment.

Packing Pointers

Suitcase Selection

♦ A small suitcase may be all you need if your travel wardrobe capsule is well planned. However, a larger 28-30" suitcase lets you lay jackets, skirts and blouses flat, with few if any folds. That means fewer wrinkles when you arrive. A waterproof suitcase will insure that your items are not damaged by anything that might leak out from other suitcases.

♦ A structured nylon hanging bag (that folds to carry) is another choice. Hang blouse and jacket on one hanger that will also hold a skirt or pant. Fold dresses over a hanger and pin at the waist.

♦ Lightweight, collapsible luggage carts and suitcases with built-in wheels save aching backs when porters are hard to find.

♦ Remove all previous routing tags before checking your luggage. And double check the new tags to be sure your suitcases are headed to the same city you are.

♦ ALWAYS have name tags both inside and outside your bags.

♦ Mark a nondescript bag with distinctive colored tags or decorative tape so you can recognize it easily and so nobody else will mistake it for theirs.

Pack Like a Pro

- Always pack well ahead of departure time and make a complete checklist. Take the list along in case your bags are lost. And use it to be sure you pack everything for the return trip too.

- Pack valuables, medications and fresh undies in your carry-on bag...just in case.

- Pack heavy items like shoes at the hinged end of the suitcase. Non-crushables like lingerie and sweaters go next, and easily wrinkled items on top.

- Keep wrinkles to a minimum by packing garments on their own hangers and in plastic cleaners' bags. Stuff tissue paper into jacket sleeves to retain shape. The hangers make unpacking a breeze, too.

- To pack pants, leave the legs hanging over the side of the suitcase while you pack other clothes on top. Then fold the legs over the top when the suitcase is full. Handle dresses the same way.

- Alternate the direction of necklines and bottoms as you layer blouses and jackets.

- Pack your robe and slippers on top, so you can put them on first and finish unpacking in cozy comfort.

Twelve Tips & Tidbits

1. Clear zip-top bags are packing lifesavers. The 10" x 12" size is the most versatile. Pack bras and panties in one, nylons in one, scarves in another and so on. Carry extras for damp swimsuits and dirty laundry.

2. Pack each shoe in its own cloth bag to prevent soiling clothes. Individual bags tuck into smaller spaces than bags made to hold a pair.

3. Keep shoes in shape by stuffing the toes with tissue paper or small items like socks.

4. Place firm leather belts around the inner edge of the suitcase. Roll softer ones and tuck into corners.

5. Use a plastic portable salt shaker with snap-on lid for bath powder. Try a film canister for face powder; it's also just the right size for a makeup brush.

6. Pack sample sizes of toiletries; they're ideal for travel and can be refilled with your favorite brands from at-home supplies. For liquids, flight attendants recommend empty foundation bottles, because glass doesn't swell in flight like plastic. For extra insurance, enclose the bottles in zip-top bags.

7. Take your share of free perfume samples from the cosmetics counter. The tiny vials are perfect for travel.

8. A small roll of masking tape makes a great lint brush. And use it to seal cosmetic bottles against leakage. In a pinch, it can even work to hold up a loose hem.

9. Pack a wardrobe repair kit. Include Fray Check to stop runs and Goddard's Dry Clean and Wrinkle Free spray to instantly freshen natural fiber garments. If you travel with knits, include a snag repair tool. And of course take a hand-washing soap like Woolite or Easy Wash.

10. An empty film canister or prescription bottle can hold a thimble, hand needles, a few straight pins, small safety pins and thread wrapped onto a small piece of cardboard. Small scissors are handy too.

11. A metal Band-Aid® box can hold a handy homemade first-aid kit. Stock it with whatever remedies you consistently use at home.

12. Slip the barrel of your hot curling iron into an empty cardboard tube to protect you clothing if you must pack it when it's still hot.

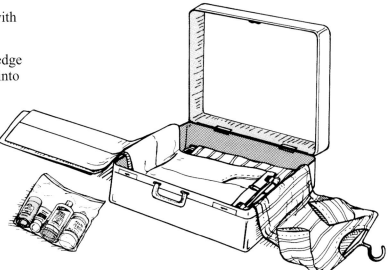

When You Arrive

♦ Give your clothes a steam bath. Remove the plastic bags (store them in your suitcase or the maid is likely to throw them away) and hang the garments from the shower-curtain rod.

Turn on the hot water (be sure the drain is open) to build up steam. Close the door tightly and in as little as 10 minutes everything will look freshly pressed.

♦ Call housekeeping to request an iron and ironing board, but don't rely on their availability. Pack a lightweight steamer or travel iron and you can always use a fluffy towel on the bathroom vanity as a substitute ironing board.

For Frequent Flyers

It's worth the investment to keep a set of travel items always packed, so you're ready at a moment's notice. Adapt this list to your personal needs:

♦ Cosmetics, toiletries and hairbrush in a cosmetic bag.

♦ Manicure set including foil-wrapped polish remover.

♦ Shower cap and disposable razors.

♦ Travel-sized blow dryer, curling iron, hot rollers.

♦ Travel iron or steamer.

♦ Extension cord; hotel outlets are never where you need them.

♦ Heating pad for achy muscles and cold rooms.

♦ Foil-wrapped spot remover.

♦ Nightie, robe, slippers.

♦ Swimsuit, leotard, lightweight jogging suit & jogging shoes.

♦ Travel alarm clock.

♦ Fold-up umbrella, sunglasses.

♦ Coffee & tea kit (cup, spoon, immersion heater, your favorite tea bags, fresh ground coffee, drip filters and cone, dehydrated soups, oatmeal).

♦ Small scissors, stapler, tape.

♦ Stationery, envelopes, stamps.

♦ Personal tape player and your favorite music or exercise tapes.

♦ Ear plugs to block out hotel noise.

Resource List

Color

- Beauty For All Seasons—Color, makeup and wardrobe consultants in most U.S. cities and many other countries. 1-800-423-3466

- Color 1—Color, makeup and wardrobe consultants in most U.S. cities and many other countries. (202) 293-9175

- Color Me Beautiful—Through Sears and JC Penney stores across the country.

Clothing

- Doncaster—Coordinated wardrobe groupings of classic styles in fine fabrics. Sold through trunk shows by individual consultants and through company studios in major cities. Sizes 2-18 and petites. 1-800-669-3662

- Trends—Fashion-forward American styling sold through trunk shows. Each style can be ordered in many fabric and color options. Sizes up to 24. (212) 869-4613

- Weekenders—Versatile, comfortable mix-and-match cotton knit separates sold through in-home presentations. (708) 465-1666

- Multiples at Home—Coordinating print and solid knitwear. Home shows by company consultants. (214) 638-3367

- Pati Palmer's designs for The McCall Pattern Company—Pattern catalogs found in most fabric stores.

Dressmakers

- Professional Association of Custom Clothiers (PACC)—National organization of highly-skilled sewing professionals with members in most major cities. P. O. Box 8476, Medford, OR 97504 (541) 772-4119

Foundation Garments

- Norvell Inc.—Custom-sized and professionally fitted bras and body shapers sold by independent representatives. (615) 529-2831 or (314) 205-0851

Swimwear

- Second Skin—Custom-designed and made-to-measure swimwear with franchise stores in many areas. 1-800-542-0136

Videos

- "Five Easy Pieces" and "Five Easy Pieces, Part 2" —Judith Rasband shows multiple examples of cluster (capsule) wardrobing using real women and their real clothes. (801) 224-1207

Seminars and Presentations

- Nancy Nix-Rice is available to present seminars and workshops on fashion, image topics and home sewing. First Impressions, 240 W. Argonne, Kirkwood, MO 63122, (314) 822-7087

Index

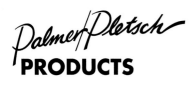

PRODUCTS

These ready-to-use, information-filled sewing how-to books, manuals and videos can be found in local book and fabric stores or ordered through Palmer/Pletsch Publishing (see address on last page).

8½ x 11 BOOKS

☐ **Looking Good**
by Nancy Nix-Rice, 160 pages, $19.95 This book provides everything women need to look their personal best—not by following what fashion dictates, but by spotlighting their best features to create the most flattering, effective look possible.

☐ **The BUSINE$$ of Teaching Sewing,** *by Marcy Miller and Pati Palmer, 128 pages, $29.95* If you want to be in the BUSINESS of teaching sewing, read this book which compiles 20 years of experience of Palmer/Pletsch, plus Miller's innovative ideas. Chapters include: Appearance and Image; Getting Started; The Lesson Plan; Class Formats; Location; Marketing, Promotion & Advertising; Pricing; Teaching Techniques; and Continuing Education—Where To Find It.

☐ **Dream Sewing Spaces—Design and Organization for Spaces Large and Small,** *by Lynette Ranney Black, 128 pages, $19.95* Make your dream a reality. Analyze your needs and your space, then learn to plan and put it together. Lots of color photos!

☐ **Couture—The Art of Fine Sewing,** *by Roberta C. Carr, 208 pages, softcover, $29.95* How-to's of couture techniques and secrets, brought to life with illustrations and dozens of garments photographed in full color.

Books are all softcover. They are also available with coil binding: $3.00 additional for large books, $2.00 for small.

☐ **The Serger Idea Book—A Collection of Inspiring Ideas from Palmer/Pletsch,** *160 pgs., $19.95* Color photos and how-to's on inspiring and fashionable ideas from the Extraordinary to the Practical.

☐ **Sewing Ultrasuede® Brand Fabrics—Ultrasuede,® Ultrasuede Light™, Caress™, Ultraleather™,** *by Marta Alto, Pati Palmer and Barbara Weiland, 128 pages, $16.95* Color photo section, plus the newest techniques to master these luxurious fabrics.

☐ **Fit for Real People**
by Marta Alto & Pati Palmer, 256 pages, $24.95 The authors write from 25 years of hands-on experience fitting thousands of people. Their practical approach is explained in their simple, logical style. Learn to finally buy the right size, then tissue fit to determine alterations. Special sections include fitting young teen girls, history of sizing, and fitting REAL people.

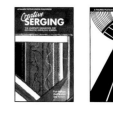
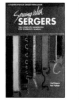
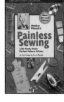

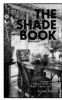
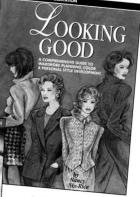
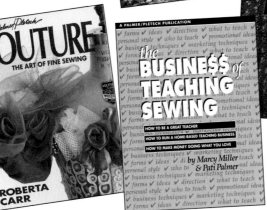

5½ x 8½ BOOKS

☐ **Sew to Success!—How to Make Money in a Home-Based Sewing Business,** *by Kathleen Spike, 128 pgs., $10.95* Learn how to establish your market, set policies and procedures, price your talents and more!

☐ **Mother Pletsch's Painless Sewing,** *NEW Revised Edition, by Pati Palmer and Susan Pletsch, 128 pgs., $8.95* The most uncomplicated sewing book of the century! Filled with sewing tips on how to sew FAST!

☐ **Sewing With Sergers—The Complete Handbook for Overlock Sewing,** *Revised Edition, by Pati Palmer and Gail Brown, 128 pages, $8.95* Learn easy threading tips, stitch types, rolled edging and flatlocking on your serger.

☐ **Creative Serging—The Complete Handbook for Decorative Overlock Sewing,** *by Pati Palmer, Gail Brown and Sue Green, 128 pages, $8.95* In-depth information and creative uses of your serger.

☐ **Sensational Silk—A Handbook for Sewing Silk and Silk-like Fabrics,** *by Gail Brown, 128 pgs., $6.95* Complete guide for sewing with silk and silkies, plus all kinds of great blouse and dress techniques.

☐ **Pants For Any Body,** *Revised Edition, by Pati Palmer and Susan Pletsch, 128 pgs., $8.95* Learn to fit pants with clear step-by-step problem and solution illustrations.

☐ **Easy, Easier, Easiest Tailoring,** *Revised Edition, by Pati Palmer and Susan Pletsch, 128 pgs., $8.95* Learn 4 different tailoring methods, easy fit tips, and timesaving machine lining.

☐ **Sew a Beautiful Wedding,** *by Gail Brown and Karen Dillon, 128 pgs., $8.95* Bridal how-to's from choosing the most flattering style to sewing with specialty fabrics.

☐ **The Shade Book,** *Revised Edition, by Judy Lindahl, 152 pages, $9.95* Learn six major shade types, variations, trimmings, hardware, hemming, care, and upkeep.

MY FIRST SEWING BOOK KITS

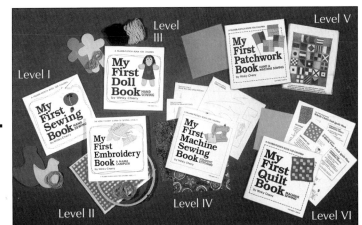

My First Sewing Books, *by Winky Cherry,* are packaged as kits with materials for a first project. Along with the Teaching Manual & Video, they offer a complete, thoroughly tested sewing program for young children. 5-to-11-year olds learn patience, manners, creativity, completion and how to follow rules...all through the enjoyment of sewing. Each book follows a project from start to finish with clever rhymes and clear illustrations. *Each book, 8½" x 8½", 40 pgs., $12.95*

☐ **My First Sewing Book** Children as young as 5 hand sew and stuff a felt bird shape. Also available in Spanish.

☐ **My First Embroidery Book** Beginners learn the importance of accuracy by making straight stitches, using a chart and gingham to make a name sampler.

☐ **My First Doll Book** Felt dolls have embroidered faces, yarn hair, and clothes. Children use the overstitch and learned in levels I and II.

☐ **My First Machine Sewing Book** With practice pages, then a fabric star, children learn about machine parts, seam allowances, tapering, snips, clips, stitching wrong sides out, and turning a shape right side out.

☐ **My First Patchwork Book** Children use a template to make a 4-square patchwork block, and can make the entire Communications Code Alphabet of patchwork flags used by sailors, soldiers, pilots and astronauts.

☐ **My First Quilt Book** Children machine stitch a quilt pieced with strips and squares, finishing it with yarn ties and, optionally, handquilted shapes.

☐ **Teaching Children to Sew Manual and Video,** *$39.95* The 112-page, 8½" x 11" **Teaching Manual,** tells you exactly how to teach young children, including preparing the environment, workshop space, class control, and the importance of incorporating other life skills along with sewing skills. In the **Video,** see Winky Cherry teach six 6-to-8 year olds how to sew in a true-life classroom setting. She introduces herself and explains the rules and shows them how to sew. Then, see close-ups of a child sewing the project in double-time. (Show this to your students.) Finally, Winky gives you a tour of an ideal classroom setup. She also talks about the tools, patterns and sewing supplies you will need. *1 hour.*

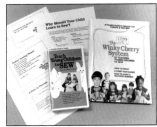

☐ **Teacher's Supply Kit,** *$49.95* The refillable kit includes these hard-to-find items—a retail value of $73.00: 50 felt pieces in assorted colors (9 x 12"), 6 colors of crochet thread on balls, 2 packs of needles with large eyes, 2 pin cushions, 12 pre-cut birds, and printed patterns for shapes.

Deluxe Kits and additional classroom materials are available. Ask for our **"As Easy As ABC"** catalog.

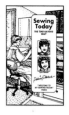

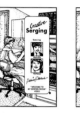

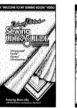
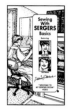
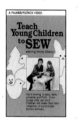

VIDEOS

According to Robbie Fanning, author and critic, "The most professional of all the (video) tapes we've seen is Pati Palmer's *Sewing Today the Time Saving Way*. This tape should serve as the standard of excellence in the field." Following that standard, we have produced 8 more videos since Time Saving! *Videos are $19.95 each.*

□ **Sewing Today the Time Saving Way,** 45 minutes featuring Lynn Raasch & Karen Dillon sharing tips and techniques to make sewing fun, fast and trouble free.

□ **Sewing to Success!,** 45 minutes featuring Kathleen Spike who presents a wealth of information on how to achieve financial freedom working in your home as a professional dressmaker.

□ **Sewing With Sergers—Basics,** 1 hour featuring Marta Alto & Pati Palmer on tensions, stitch types and their uses, serging circles, turning corners, gathering and much more.

□ **Sewing With Sergers—Advanced,** 1 hour featuring Marta Alto & Pati Palmer on in-depth how-to's for rolled edging & flatlocking as well as garment details.

□ **Creative Serging,** 1 hour featuring Marta Alto & Pati Palmer on how to use decorative threads, yarns and ribbons on your serger. PLUS: fashion shots!

□ **Creative Serging II,** 1 hour featuring Marta Alto & Pati Palmer showing more creative ideas, including in-depth creative rolled edge.

□ **Two-Hour Trousers,** 1 hour, 40 minutes, featuring Kathleen Spike with fit tips using our unique tissue-fitting techniques, the best basics, and designer details.

□ **Sewing Ultrasuede® Brand Fabrics—Ultrasuede®, Facile®, Caress™, Ultraleather™** 1 hour featuring Marta Alto & Pati Palmer with clear, step-by-step sewing demonstrations and fashion show.

□ **Creative Home Decorating Ideas: Sewing Projects for the Home,** 1 hour featuring Lynette Ranney Black showing creative, easy ideas for windows, walls, tables and more. Companion to *Creative Serging for the Home.*

Teach Young Children to Sew is part of the training package described on the previous page.

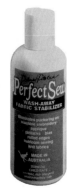

INTERFACINGS

Ask us about our new, extra-wide fusible weft **PerfectFuse™ Interfacings**. Available in four weights, they come in 1-yard packages in both black and ecru-white. Call for more information and pricing.

PALMER/PLETSCH WORKSHOPS

Our "Sewing Vacations" are offered on a variety of topics, including *Pant Fit, Fit, Tailoring, Creative Serging, Ultrasuede, Couture* and a special *Sewing Update/ Best of Palmer/Pletsch* session. Workshops are held at the new Palmer/Pletsch International Training Center near the Portland, Oregon, airport.

Teacher training sessions are also available on each topic. They include practice teaching sessions, hair styling, make-up and publicity photo session, up to 300 slides and script, camera-ready workbook handouts and publicity flyer and the manual **The BUSINE$$ of Teaching Sewing.**

Call or write for schedules and information:

Palmer/Pletsch School of Sewing
P.O. Box 12046
Portland, OR 97212
(503) 294-0696

MAIL-ORDER INFORMATION ON McCALL'S BASIC DRESS FIT PATTERN BY PALMER/PLETSCH

All pattern company basic fit patterns, except McCall's, are available in local fabric stores.

You can order McCall's through a fabric store that carries McCall's. If there isn't one in your area, call 800/255-2762 or fax 913/776-0200. Have a credit card ready. Palmer/Pletsch instructors provide this pattern in fit classes.

Palmer/Pletsch also carries a Trends bulletin on Knitting Machines, plus hard-to-find and unique notions including Perfect Sew Wash-Away Fabric Stabilizer, Perfect Sew Needle Threader and decorative serging threads. Check your local fabric store or contact Palmer/Pletsch Publishing, P.O. Box 12046, Portland, OR 97212-0046. (503) 274-0687 or 1-800-728-3784 (order desk).

160